Leadership Skills for Health and Social Care Professionals

Annie Phillips
Writer on Health and Health Management
Specialist Paediatric Speech and Language Therapist,
Somerset Partnership

Foreword by

Pam Enderby MBE, PhD, FRCSLT
Professor of Community Rehabilitation,
University of Sheffield

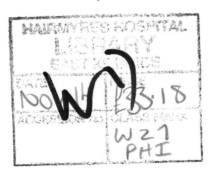
Radcliffe Publishing
London • New York

Radcliffe Publishing Ltd
33–41 Dallington Street
London
EC1V 0BB
United Kingdom

www.radcliffehealth.com

British Library Cataloguing in Publication Data

A catalogue record for this book is available from the British Library.

ISBN-13: 978 184619 883 0

The paper used for the text pages of this book is FSC® certified. FSC (The Forest Stewardship Council®) is an international network to promote responsible management of the world's forests.

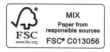

Typeset by Phoenix Photosetting, Chatham, Kent
Printed and bound by TJ International Ltd, Padstow, Cornwall

Contents

Foreword

The many and significant changes to international health, education and social care systems over the past few years are likely to continue as countries are faced with the challenges of financial restrictions at the same time as the need for expanding health and social care structures. This in response to increasing numbers of children with significant disabilities surviving longer, the needs of the more elderly population, greater expectations and rapidly changing technology. All of these will have a substantial impact on the technical and personal skills required by allied health professionals.

One thing is certain. All those involved in health, education and social care will see substantial changes during their time employed within their profession. They will need continually to consider and amend their contribution, develop their skills and respond to new knowledge and technology in order to collaborate effectively in different settings and to meet the changing needs. This will require professional confidence and competence of a different style and nature from what has been required before. More individuals will be working independently, without the security of a prescribed management structure; many will be working with and responsible for assistants and volunteers. They will need to ensure that they comply with the professional standards set by the regulatory authorities and legislative structure. This demands a greater emphasis on clarity of communication, explicit awareness of competence and the confidence to assert one's knowledge, as well as a surety of one's limitations.

This book will help professionals to develop their leadership skills in order to equip them for the changing world and manage the many demands and stresses in a positive and productive manner. The objective of the book is that readers will increase their competence and confidence, which will be of benefit to themselves, their colleagues and, most importantly, their clients.

Pam Enderby MBE, PhD, FRCSLT
Professor of Community Rehabilitation, University of Sheffield
June 2013

About the author

Annie Phillips has written professionally about health and health management since she qualified as a speech and language therapist in 1978. She has over 30 years' NHS experience in primary and secondary care as a clinician and manager.

Her first 10 years as a speech and language therapist, specialising in adult neurology and elderly care, led to the research and publication of an international dysphasia/dementia screening test, presented at the 1986 British Aphasiology Conference. She has won various prizes and awards for her subsequent work, and in the 1990s was a finalist in the Medeconomics Good Management Awards and regional winner in a national British Institute of Management competition on Change Management.

She worked as a practice and fund manager for a five-partner training GP practice in central Brighton from 1989 to 1998; from then as an independent health advisor, trainer and management consultant to general practice and PCTs. As a management consultant, her interest focused on organisational analysis and the development of healthy organisations, with an emphasis on finding ways to manage stresses and conflicts, understanding and alleviating dysfunctional communication and developing effective management strategies.

In 2000, she returned to clinical work as a paediatric speech and language therapist, and continues in this work to date.

Throughout her career she has written extensively for the therapy, medical and management press on contemporary management issues for a range of publications, including *Health Service Journal*, *Community Care*, *Pulse*, *Medi-Economics*, *Doctor*, *Primary Care Manager* and Croner Publications, with a focus on healthcare politics and clinical management. Her first book, *The Business Planning Toolkit: a workbook for the primary care team*, was published in 2002 (Radcliffe Publishing), and was swiftly followed by three others, including the sister volume to this book, *Developing Assertiveness Skills for Health and Social Care Professionals*.

Annie can be contacted via the publishers.

Acknowledgements

Thanks to all those of my family and friends who have supported me in my own personal development: all my favourite people (you know who you are!). Your love, friendship, support and ideas have sustained me over the years.

I also wish to record my thanks and debt of gratitude to Dr Pam Enderby, whom I met first in the early 1980s, and whose work inspired me to begin thinking about the importance of evidence-based working; and subsequently the partners at St Peter's Medical Centre, Brighton – especially Dr Howard Carter – for the help, encouragement and valuable advice gained during my employment through the 1990s. On to all my PCT, training and management colleagues – some of whom were inspirational; all of whom challenged my thinking. Without all of these people, my journey into understanding the theory of clinical management would not have been possible. It is in these jobs that I really learned that management was a professional field in its own right, with academic rigour, and not simply an add-on to clinical work.

And on to this decade, to those colleagues too numerous to mention whose wise counsel challenges me to continue learning – including all those who continue to teach me as I work with them, the current bunch being the Somerset Integrated Therapy Team, especially – but not exclusively – my dear friends Tash, Lyndsey and Lauren, and for the management team who tirelessly support me in my process! Special thanks to Fanny Rowe, whose devolved management style and expert leadership allow us therapists to feel safe, while encouraging and supporting our creativity and developing clinical skills.

I want to thank all those whose thoughts and ideas have, over the years, found their way into my subconscious, so they are now indistinguishable from my own. In this vein, if I have unintentionally misquoted anyone, my apologies. I have attempted to give sources of work where possible, but apologise if, inadvertently, I have failed to record it correctly. Should you note any queries, errors or omissions, please contact the publisher. Special thanks too to my editors, Jamie Etherington and Elisabeth Doyle, for all their hard work and for dealing so sensitively with any changes required; and finally to the typesetters, Phoenix Photosetting, for making the book look fabulous.

Finally, my very special thanks as always to my partner Lin, for her love, encouragement and support; for her thoughtful additions, insightful editing; and for gracefully giving me the time out from our family commitments to continue writing.

Introduction

This book was written as a sister volume to my first book, *Developing Assertiveness Skills for Health and Social Care Professionals*, which invites the reader to explore the advantages of using assertiveness as the main tool of effective, advanced communication skills in health or social care settings and in their dealings with people. This book takes us one step beyond, taking a broad look at the interpersonal communication skills required to communicate more effectively, and applying assertiveness skills in developing the reader's professional and leadership qualities. My reader is anyone who works in the public or private sector as a clinician or a manager: anyone who deals with people – colleagues, staff, the public – on a daily basis, and needs these dealings to be thoughtful, effective and stress free. The target market is all those who work in care or medical settings: acute medicine, primary care and the community; any member of the healthcare team, with or without a management role, who wants to understand how to develop their relationships with their colleagues and managers. Anyone who needs to:
➤ understand and alleviate barriers to effective communication
➤ manage stresses and conflicts
➤ develop effective supervisory, people and management skills.

The recently published draft report from the Commission on Improving Dignity in Care for Older People (2012) has prompted reflections and discussions on professionalism across the healthcare workforce. We are debating what goes wrong, how to right it, the need to behave in a professional way, what professionalism looks like. The Health Professions Council has identified 'treating patients and service users with respect, communicating clearly, involving people in decisions about their own care, keeping accurate records of treatments and interventions' as fundamental to good professional practice.[1]

---

1 Health Professions Council. *Fitness to Practise Annual Report 2008* and *Standards of Conduct, Performance and Ethics 2008*. Also: Health Professions Council. *Professionalism in Nursing, Midwifery and the Allied Health Professions in Scotland: a report to the coordinating council for the NMAHP Contribution to the Healthcare Quality Strategy for NHS Scotland*. Health Professions Council; 2012.

These have been reported on recently, and I want this book to contribute to the debate and help to sharpen up ideas of professionalism in healthcare.

Here, we target information about the broader aspects of communication – understanding ourselves and others, our motivations, interests and perspectives – to encourage the development of interpersonal skills, and to keep our observational and caring skills sharp. All of us working in the caring professions should keep in mind a need to work with intellectual rigour, emotional intelligence and compassion, and should apply these qualities in all our dealings, be it with patients or staff. We should be able to recognise, support and empathise with distress, foster feelings of warmth and kindness, develop qualities of patience and tolerance, and look critically at difficulties in order to learn from them and develop wisdom.

The book begins with a refresher on assertiveness skills, then moves into the personal skills needed to navigate successfully through a career in the caring professions. The book challenges the reader to reconstruct their communication and behave more confidently and equally. It provokes and encourages the reader to invest in their own personal and professional development. I analyse some of the barriers to good communication, and the management and clinical skills we need to develop professionally: confidence, self-awareness and development of critical faculties. The book is an essential tool for all health and social care workers aiming to understand more about how manage themselves and their communication partners: their colleagues in health, education, social services, local government. There is an implicit assumption that we are working towards an integrated model of working across all sectors, hence the need to look at communicating in organisations and understanding another's perspective.

The book is divided into four sections. The first section summarises basic assertiveness skills, and how to apply these in difficult situations, including information on giving constructive, kindly and clear feedback to staff in challenging circumstances, and managing conflict and disputes. There is an overview on some of the skills of negotiation, making and refusing requests, managing conflict and aggression.

In Section 2, we begin to move forward, and explore how to use assertion skills to develop professionally and personally. We address the foundations of good communication and the need to understand what our own organisation and team really looks like. We begin to develop an understanding of ourselves and others: our need to be assertive, our motivations, our personality, how we work within a team and within the broader health and social care settings. I include information on leadership skills, facilitating, culture and leadership, and how best to communicate with our stakeholders.

In Section 3, we explore the development of personal management skills: how to delegate and how to give constructive, clear feedback to staff in appraisal, interviewing and disciplinary procedures, developing supervision and support skills.

Finally, in Section 4 we learn how to apply some of the learned skills into common work situations: strategies for improving personal communication and organisation. We look at using assertiveness in planning and managing life to help make it stress free through goal setting and time and change management.

At the end of each chapter I have included some summary points, which should assist the reader in reflecting on the concepts explored and identifying any learning needs.

Confident people achieve success as they bring themselves into the best focus possible. They take control of situations. They take responsibility to use all their capabilities. They do not avoid conflict or difficulties or ignore problems. They take charge and confront inefficiency, unfairness, mediocrity or poor conduct with honesty and clarity, without which they could not achieve in life or work. Assertive people face their insecurities, and learn how to cope with authority. They allow themselves to make mistakes, knowing that assurance comes with experience. They know there is no such thing as perfection in people, remembering that good intentions are as important as any other quality. They listen, ask questions, take advice and then act. Successful people do not leave anything to chance: they take charge of their life. This is the book that teaches you how to develop those skills.

Annie Phillips
June 2013

Section 1

Assertiveness skills

CHAPTER 1

Why is assertiveness important?

All of us have the right to be treated with respect, to be listened to and taken seriously. We have the rights to set our own priorities and to choose for ourselves. We have the right to express our own feelings and opinions without fear. We have the right to make mistakes.

These rights are important at a personal and professional level, but crucial to anyone developing leadership skills, when the expectations are higher and our need to communicate well in a highly complex and demanding work context such as health and social care is even more important. Behaving assertively helps us to take charge and acts in ways that invite respect, accepting our own limitations and strengths, leading to clearer communication.

Assertive skills alone enable us to fulfil our clinical or management roles in any integrated health or social care setting more effectively, and to cope more readily with feelings of frustration or inadequacy. This book takes us one step beyond, taking a broad look at the range of interpersonal communication skills required to communicate at a higher level, developing the reader's professional or leadership qualities. Anyone who works in either the public or private sector as clinician or manager, anyone who deals with people – colleagues, senior staff, the public – on a daily basis, and needs these dealings to be thoughtful, effective and stress free, will benefit.

To be assertive does not mean you will always get what you want, or that all your problems will be solved. It is one tool among many. Assertive techniques help us to communicate in constructive and satisfying ways, to achieve workable results in difficult situations, and can assist in resolving conflicts without aggression. These are essential techniques to understand and use in all our work roles.

Assertiveness is a skill that is particularly important for women. Women make up the majority of workers in the caring professions; and they are much more likely than men to put themselves last, and can therefore find it harder to communicate their own needs or to develop themselves or their career. There are some noticeable gender differences. Both sexes draw constantly on their emotional and intellectual resources when dealing with clinical and managerial conflicts, and struggle to provide a good service with limited resources and sometimes little peer group support. Women, however, are more likely to feel guilty when they do not, or are unable to, live up to the caring image. Women are socialised to want to be thought of as indispensable: the work can involve sacrifice; we find it hard to delegate and certainly do not want to offend. Although men generally find it easier to be assertive, some find it harder to develop the fine-tuned and complex verbal and non-verbal skills needed to listen and communicate with empathy, sympathy and focus. They sometimes tend towards aggression rather than passivity, and may struggle to rein in or understand their own emotional responses if they have not been socialised to do so. Thus, generally, more women than men seek ways to become more assertive.

In teaching assertiveness, I like to think we are looking at behaving with good intent, and integrity, with the motivation to care for others and ourselves, being kind and thoughtful in the ways we conduct ourselves at work, paying attention to ourselves and others in a focused, compassionate way. It is important that we are motivated to behave with understanding and tolerance, and this in turn helps to generate and feed our own, and other people's, good feelings. Compassion requires thoughtfulness, curiosity and openness, and it also at times requires courage – and these are qualities that we all at times struggle with. We have to be brave to be assertive.

Thus, used well, assertiveness is not about behaving selfishly, but rather about using our skills of attention, reasoning, awareness of feeling and behaviour to build the attributes of sensitivity, sympathy, empathy, non-judgement, care, and compassion for others and ourselves. The assertive person recognises their own limits and is able to call a halt before they burn out. They give themselves time to rest and replenish their energies, and recognise that their needs are no more or no less than others, but equal.

SOME OF THE SITUATIONS THAT ASSERTIVE BEHAVIOUR CAN HELP WITH

➤ Complex communication: conflict, manipulation, aggression.
➤ Time management.
➤ Identification of obstacles to career or personal development.
➤ Overcoming work and people demands.
➤ Making and refusing requests.
➤ Handling criticism and compliments.
➤ Coping with rejection, building self-esteem.
➤ Giving constructive criticism.
➤ Staff appraisals and disciplinary procedures.
➤ Negotiating.
➤ Goal setting.

Behaving assertively helps us to communicate directly and powerfully at work; and can also defend against aggression or defensive behaviour when hopes and plans are thwarted. Negotiation and compromise form the lynchpin in assertiveness training. The assertive person takes charge and acts in ways that invite respect. This in turn leads to clearer communication, and any potential confusion or discord is alleviated.

There are many unusual management situations in the private and statutory healthcare sector: senior practitioners and clinical managers who are torn in many ways, balancing the demands of their staff with those of clients/patients and managers, needing to uphold professional standards while acknowledging financial pressures and the needs of the service overall; GPs, who now have to balance their professional and commissioning role; practice managers, unique in their role as representatives of general practice, acting as advocates for the staff and patients, leading and yet in turn 'managed' by their employers, the GPs, clinicians and the practitioners, all of whom have to find the very best for those they help while working to the management and government agenda, balancing personal and professional needs, and managing tensions – what is best for the client within the resources available? These unusual and diverse relationships can cause conflict. Assertiveness skills enable us to see our role more clearly and cope more readily with feelings of frustration or inadequacy. We need to be able, too, to express anger, frustrations and anxiety constructively in order to prevent further stress, improve management and improve services.

Eric Berne[1] was one of the first psychologists to identify behavioural traits in communicating which impacted on the success of the communication. His term for what we would now call assertiveness was 'adult': the assertive response is 'in adult': a neutral and fair communication style.

A quick checklist may show you what your most usual behavioural traits are, and therefore give you some indication of your need to learn some assertiveness skills.
➤ Do you see yourself as someone who is *passive*? Avoiding conflict, a victim?
➤ Or *aggressive*, angry, defensive, and competitive?
➤ *Manipulative*? Someone who behaves in devious ways, appearing to think highly of others but with an undercurrent of disapproval.
➤ The *assertive* person, however, says what they want, respectfully, without resorting to anger or manipulation; they take responsibility for themselves, their needs, feelings and reactions.

We are all a mix of behavioural styles, and our history and genes dictate our personality traits to some extent, but it is possible to communicate more honestly, openly and directly, and avoid the manipulation, anger and passivity that may be a more habitual stance.

---

1 Berne E. *Games People Play*. Penguin Books; 1968.

Assertiveness is especially relevant for us as workers in the caring sector, because we do care: we care inherently for the people we work with and for, and our organisation. We can therefore feel very guilty when we do not, or are unable to, live up to the caring image. We often think of ourselves as indispensable: our work can involve sacrifice; we often find it hard to delegate. We do not want to offend. It is extremely easy for us to feel guilty. Consider the following scenarios:

> you feel guilty about keeping to time boundaries – you need to be available to your patients/clients and colleagues at all times

> you do not move to a more stimulating or rewarding job because you know there will be difficulties recruiting your replacement

> you do not push your staff as hard as you should because you can empathise with their difficulties around increasing public demands

> you reluctantly accept a new system of working that you have reservations about because you do not want to offend the colleagues/your manager, who are enthusiastic about it.

Anyone who consistently behaves in this way will overstretch and exhaust themselves. They are taking care of everyone else but themselves, at huge cost to their own physical and mental well-being. They think themselves indispensible, and soon 'burn out'.

Here is a useful exercise to do with a friend or sympathetic colleague.

EXERCISE 1

The compassion trap

Using the columns below, list those things that you do for other people because they ask you, not because you want to do them or accept that they are part of your role.

Work	Friendships	Home

For example:

Work	Friendships	Home
Always make the tea	Always arrange family gatherings	Do majority of the housework
Work overtime almost every day, unpaid	Talk with X for hours on end even through I have other family demands	Go to parent's evening every time
Take the on call every Christmas		

➤ Swap lists.
➤ Role play the situation. Your part is to say 'no', politely but firmly.
➤ What does the 'no' feel like?

If you feel you need more practice, read Chapter 7, Making and refusing requests, in my sister book, *Developing Assertiveness Skills for Health and Social Care Professionals*.

HOW TO CHANGE

To be assertive is not to behave selfishly; it is about responsible self-care. The assertive person recognises their own limits, manages their own resources so as to work effectively, without resentment, and is able to call a halt before they burn out. They give themselves time to rest and replenish their energies, so that when they do give once more they do so with sustainable strength and enthusiasm.

If you find delegation difficult, assume responsibility for other people's needs or find it easier to make decisions for friends, family and co-workers, you are taking inappropriate responsibility for others' lives. Women in particular are reluctant to relinquish work-based power, as it can be one of the only areas of their life where they hold power. If this is the case, by taking more power for yourself assertively you will feel able to give up this strong manipulative hold and claim real equality. You will still be able to show compassion, love and care to others; but the choice will be yours; you are not compelled always to put others' needs before your own to maintain your own self-worth.

YOUR RIGHTS

When we acknowledge that we too have certain rights, we set ourselves free from the dependence on others for their approval.

Consider the following.

Sara is a successful and respected duty social work manager. She pioneered a departmental move, and the development of some new, innovative services. She has acted as the catalyst for a lot of positive change. After much consideration, she has decided that she wishes to resign and move on, after only 18 months in the post.

Her employers ask why she is leaving; they are concerned that the department will collapse without her. Sara feels caught in a trap. She is concerned that she will appear selfish if she leaves so soon. Perhaps she should carry on for another few years. She feels guilt and sympathy for her colleagues, left to manage 'by themselves'. Eventually she states her position assertively. She acknowledges the department's position, and explains that she has enjoyed bringing in the innovations that she has and that she has contributed and learned a lot. However, she wants to develop other skills now, that she feels are better suited to another role. The others hear her and respect her clarity and decision; she herself leaves feeling satisfied that she has made the right choice.

The explanation Sara gave to her colleagues demonstrated her professional concern, but also showed them that she too had needs and other plans that she wished to fulfil. She chose for herself assertively.

We all have the right to set our own priorities and to choose for ourselves. We have the right to express our own feelings and opinions – including saying 'no' – without fear. We have the right to make mistakes.

Examine these rights in more detail. What do they mean for us?

1   We have the right to be treated with respect

In any system where power inequalities are regarded as natural, this is hard. This culture only works for those in the most senior position. Within this system it is very difficult for lower grade staff to have and to offer opinions. It is easy to forget that what we feel and what we have to say as an intelligent and informed individual counts as there is always someone ready and willing to put you in your place. We need to remember in these circumstances that our own needs and opinions matter too. Being treated with respect means being noticed. Others may not agree with what you have to say, but you have a right to a voice and may be able to offer a valuable additional perspective. Remember that your time is valued and appreciated: for example, people cannot always assume that they can talk with you at *their* convenience.

2   We have the right to set our own priorities

If you are feeling disempowered, it is very easy to let others lead your agenda. Begin to see yourself as someone who deserves as much time, effort and energy as your family, your colleagues, the organisation and those you help. If you permit yourself the right to look after your own life, the need for others to speak *for* you is removed.

Let us take another example.

Kate is a practice manager who has allocated some time in her day to review the practice accounts. The practice is busy dealing with a flu epidemic, but among other pressures and deadlines, Kate has to review these accounts before a meeting with the accountant the following day. She wants to present a summary to the senior partner at their lunchtime review. When she arrives in her office, one of the partners rushes in to greet her in a panic. He asks her if she could possibly cover reception, as they are short – and it is a Monday morning. Kate acknowledges the partner's difficulties, but reasserts her need and wish to continue with the work she is doing. She will, however, do her utmost to obtain locum cover, and picks up the phone instantly to set this in motion. Kate, as a fellow professional, has set her own limits and priorities for the day; she need not allow the senior partner to organise her, as she is capable of organising herself.

3 We have the right to ask for what we want

Here you establish your right to identify and communicate your needs as an equal. It is easy, especially when you are newly qualified or new to an organisation, to feel that you do not matter, and to be in awe of others who seem much older and more experienced. All of us need to remember that we too have the right to ask for what we want, and to ask for information or clarification if we do not understand.

➤ Allow yourself to communicate your needs to others, remembering of course that you cannot always expect those needs to be met – allow yourself room for negotiation.

➤ Never accept substandard accommodation to work in. Everyone working in the public sector is entitled to accommodation that is quiet, free from distractions and suitably furnished. Refuse to work in unsuitable premises. It is only by doing this that some respect will eventually be shown to you and your profession.

➤ Never allow yourself to accept rude, aggressive or undermining behaviour.

➤ If you do not voice your concerns, your work will be undervalued.

➤ Ask for what you want – you have nothing to lose. If you do not ask, others will not know.

4 We have the right to be listened to and taken seriously

What you say may not, of course, always be right, but you do have a right to air your opinions. Do not allow your age or (apparent) lack of professional standing to belittle you.

5 We have the right to set our own goals

Make your own choices when decisions need to be made, and set your own goals, your own standards and limits.

6 We have the right to say 'no' without feeling guilty

Make your own decisions and choices, which includes saying 'no' periodically to demands made on you. If you are being asked to do something that you feel unable or unwilling to do, think again before automatically agreeing.

7 We have the right to express our own feelings and opinions

You have the right to hold an opinion, to have feelings and emotions about issues, and to express them appropriately. Do not allow others to deny you your feelings. Be ready to stand by your own opinions when others try to belittle you. Do not automatically concede to preserve the peace, or aggressively present opinions dogmatically, denying others the right to share theirs. The assertive person respects another's opinions and feelings, while acknowledging that she or he holds a (possibly) differing view.

8   We have the right to make mistakes

Acknowledge the mistake and start afresh. In this way your self-esteem and confidence in yourself is retained. Take responsibility for your own decisions and deal with the consequences. This may also show flexibility and that your thinking has advanced.

9   We have the right to ask for and get information from professionals

Remember your individual, or consumer, rights when faced with professionals, who often withhold information to retain power or authority. Do not be afraid to admit that you do not understand, as often an acknowledgement of your own weaknesses will be met with sympathy and respect. Admit to ignorance or confusion, to not knowing, and feel confident to ask for clarification or more information. Ask clearly and confidently; avoiding subtleties and suggestions. A clear, direct question should be met with an equally clear, respectful response.

10   We have the right to receive criticism in our own way

Allow yourself the right to accept criticism if you feel that it is fair, but ask for clarification or example if you feel the criticism is unjustified.

11   We have the right to get what we pay for

You have a right to reflect that you deserve fair treatment from people whose services you have requested. If you attend a course that you feel was poor value for money, say so! If your client takes phone calls throughout your appointment, air your grievance! You deserve better treatment.

12   We have the right to choose for ourselves

The assertive person successfully assesses his or her own behaviour and thus releases him- or herself from dependence on the opinions of others. We have the right to chose whether or not to get involved, to chose privacy, to be assertive.

EXERCISE 2

List your own needs, the favourite things in your life that you enjoy, in the left hand column.

For example, I like watching daytime TV/I like living alone/I like reading in bed. In the right column, list any people who impose on those activities and say why you feel you are unable to do the activity.

I like eating lunch alone	*There is pressure on me to eat with the team in the staffroom*

You can also chose when, where and if you wish to be assertive. Do not berate yourself if you cannot, or chose not to, do so.

SOME BLOCKS TO ASSERTIVENESS

What prevents people from being assertive? Many people are anxious about acquiring a new skill or may procrastinate. Others are frightened. They may have a fear of rejection, of hurting others, of violence, of failure or of financial insecurity (people are less assertive and more compliant in an economic downturn, when they may fear losing their job). There may be few assertive role models around; there may be a lack of opportunity to see and acquire the skills. For some, they may have cultural, philosophical or religious beliefs that prevent an interest – assertive behaviour can be seen as threatening or selfish in some cultures. If you have emotional blocks such as those above, try questioning these, and imagine the real consequences of behaving assertively.

Remember that to be assertive is also to behave compassionately: thoughtfully, with curiosity and openness; and courageously.

KEY POINTS

➤ Behaving assertively helps at both a professional and a personal level.
➤ The assertive person takes charge and acts in ways that invite respect, accepting their own limitations and strengths, leading to clearer communication.
➤ Learning to be assertive is seen as an important component in cognitive-behavioural approaches to tackling anger, anxiety, depression and poor self-esteem.
➤ In assertiveness, it is important that we are motivated to behave with good intent, kindness, tolerance and compassion.
➤ The assertive person recognises that their needs are no more and no less than others, but equal.

➤ Assertive skills enable us to see our role in the caring professions more clearly and to cope more readily with feelings of frustration or inadequacy.

➤ To be assertive does not mean you will always get what you want, or that all your problems will be solved. Assertiveness is one tool among many.

➤ All of us have the right to be treated with respect, to be listened to and taken seriously. We have the right to set our own priorities and to choose for ourselves. We have the right to express our own feelings and opinions without fear. We have the right to make mistakes.

➤ Compassion requires thoughtfulness, curiosity and openness, and it also at times requires courage – and these are qualities that we all at times struggle with. Sometimes we have to be brave to be assertive.

FURTHER READING

Both Anne Dickson and Gail Lindenfield's books on assertiveness, self-esteem and confidence building are excellent, and accessible.

Dickson A. *Difficult Conversations: what to say in tricky situations without ruining the relationship*. New ed. Piatkus; 2006.

Dickson A. *The Mirror Within: a new look at sexuality*. Quartet Books; 1985.

Lindenfield G. *Assert Yourself: simple steps to getting what you want*. Thorsons; 2001.

Lindenfield G. *Self Esteem: simple steps to develop self-worth and heal emotional wounds*. Thorsons; 2000.

Lindenfield G. *Super Confidence: simple steps to build self-assurance*. Thorsons; 2000.

Women and assertiveness

Women in particular need to develop assertiveness skills. Men, for various physiological, psychological, socio-cultural and contextual reasons, find it easier to assert themselves in the workplace. For more information about women and assertiveness, *see* Chapter 2 in my sister book, *Developing Assertiveness Skills for Health and Social Care Professionals*.

The fact remains that, over the years, there has been little change in gender stereotyping, both in and out of work. Masculine characteristics are deemed to be assertiveness, independence, power and self-reliance, and feminine characteristics are traditionally caring, helpfulness and sharing. The stereotypes are common in many cultures, and there can be a backlash if you act out of role. Success at work is usually associated with the male traits of aggression, emotional stability and rationality. If women manifest these behaviours, the fear is that they will be seen as tough, hard, unlikable. There is a penalty for women behaving counter to stereotypical expectations, at a cost to success. However, although women more than men can face difficulties when they behave assertively (as it can be perceived as unexpected/unusual behaviour), there are ways we can work with the behaviour to achieve advantage and acceptability.

Women tend to operate through guile, passive-aggressive wheedling and manipulation instead of communicating cleanly and honestly.[1] Women need to learn to develop their egos: to be prouder of themselves and their success. They can learn symbolically to 'take more space' for themselves, by altering their body language and verbal skills to support a stronger sense of self.

This is not to say that any of us women should give up our well-developed attributes of compassion and being empathetic, but that we can learn to understand why and what we feel, and begin to tolerate these emotions. Many men too, who are hard-wired differently, would benefit from learning how to develop skills of empathy, compassionate attention and good listening.

If we deny our own needs and wishes at the expense of others, we make ourselves available to others to our own detriment, and, ultimately, others'

---

1 Simmonds R. *The Curse of the Good Girl*. Penguin; 2009.

too. Our compassion traps us, which is why it is important to harness some assertiveness skills.

We all have needs, rights, opinions and choices that we have a right to exercise. Because of cultural pressures, women in particular find it difficult to acknowledge these needs and rights, and to own them. Society and patriarchal culture has shaped all of us, and there are gender-specific roles and expectations that play out. Men and women clearly differ in their life experience, in their presentation and socialisation. The roles men and women play out have an impact on how they feel about themselves, their value and their role in the world. A bigger role in the outer world makes us more assertive, more confident, gives us higher self-esteem.

➤ Think for a moment how men and women differ in their life experience, in their presentation, socialisation. What opportunities exist for both?
➤ What are the current stereotypical preferences in life roles at home, work? Think of yourself, your parents, people you know. Who does the main bulk of the childcare? The school run? The housework? Are certain roles gender-aligned?
➤ How did/do men and women behave differently with girl and boy babies – in their choice of clothes, games, toys, play? Which play is outward looking, physically challenging, and which is more inward-focussed, more nurturing?
➤ On a scale of 1 to 10, how socially confidant as a woman do you feel, at work, and out and about?

We know that gender and culture differences mean that things said one way are interpreted differently by others. There are differences in the way men and women vie for power, for status and connection in their communication styles. If we explore some of these differences and their impact on the ways men and women communicate, together and with each other, we can see how this affects our ability to be assertive.

EXERCISE 1

What follows are some commonly used female discourse patterns. Mark any that you feel are common to you.

Female discourse patterns

➤ To believe, and say, they have got it wrong.
➤ Indirectness.
➤ Happy with silence.
➤ Raising topics of interest to listener.
➤ Low confidence/aggression.

➤ Frequent apologies.
➤ Asking lots of questions to gain information and understand the other person.
➤ More likely to adapt to the style of speaker.
➤ Waiting for turn to come before speaking.
➤ Smiling more.
➤ Non-verbal attentiveness ('silent applause'): listening, observing, quiet, sympathetic approach.
➤ More deferential, keeping quiet about their successes.
➤ Asking men what interests them, and listening.
➤ Better at reciprocal communication, keeping the flow going between both parties, taking turns.
➤ Communicating with less certainty, confidence, diffident but with more respect for feelings: 'This might seem a silly question but …', 'You've probably thought of this before, but …'
➤ Apologising, taking blame, admitting ignorance.
➤ Using an attenuated/personal voice: 'I'm intrigued by your comment/can you say a bit more?'
➤ More likely to back off if are interrupted, less likely to persist.
➤ Building on others' questions, asking questions to elicit ideas.
➤ Tentative communication: speaking with low confidence/aggression: no boasting/bragging, downplaying their own authority.
➤ Seeking agreement before changing topics: '… shall we look at X now?'
➤ Avoiding stating they have revised/planned activity/schedule – feeling discomfort with power.
➤ Agreeing, supporting, encouraging: making suggestions not commanding.
➤ More likely to adapt to the style of speaker.

DEVELOP A PROFESSIONAL IMAGE

Take an honest look at how you present: the more feminine your image, the more female your presentation, the less seriously you will be taken professionally. Remember that confidence and high self-esteem are indicated when you no longer need to conform to someone else's standard, so find your own style, which may be to be quieter and less assuming, but efficient.

➤ Authority or seniority is usually understated, with clothing simple and formal.
➤ You will show more authority if you stand face to face with someone, rather than you sitting and they standing; lower the pitch of your voice, and slightly increase the volume.
➤ Check your body language: make sure you look the person in the eye, as you say 'no', or try moving away or making a 'no' hand movement.

➤ Check that you are not smiling apologetically as you talk, maintain firm eye contact, sit or stand upright, and keep your voice steady and clear.

➤ Self-publicise to build your confidence: take credit for your achievements, do not assume your accomplishments are routine.

➤ Let other people's opinions of you do the talking, as in: 'I was asked to make the key speech at the conference this year' or 'I'll be tied up next week: I'm heading the new clinical governance project'.

➤ Angle your stories to highlight any assertive qualities: 'I negotiated my way through that situation, and we both achieved outcomes we were happy with.'

Even today, many men have only known women as subordinates. No matter how knowledgeable and skilled, female clinicians and managers may still be perceived as flirtatious, competitive, too warm or too hard. Some men feel a loss of identity; they feel invaded, insecure and threatened by competent women. These men need to be educated to become better 'process' observers. They fail to perceive emotional cues and need to learn to respond with understanding in the same way. Women can assist by continuous determination for a professional relationship – mutual help, information-sharing and socialisation. As we model good professional and management behaviour, we break down prejudices and help men to form new expectations of us.

Women's advantage is our well-developed communication skills – we are more able at developing and maintaining communication links, more capable of building reciprocal relationships, very good at process observation, trained to pick up other's discomforts, anxieties, fears and angers, and able to respond to emotions instinctively. An impressive list, and one that lends us to learning to be more assertive. However, because of these skills, women also often say much more about the way they feel than they then feel comfortable with.

We need to remember that we too are intelligent, capable and equal human beings, especially when we feel undermined by our imperialist medical system that assumes medics, and men in particular, hold the power. Health and social care are hierarchical organisations, with unwritten rules at play; the medics and those in senior positions dominate the hierarchy, which leaves women managers, in particular, in a much less powerful position.

This is shifting, as those in less powerful positions are gaining more confidence and authority to question the medical ascendancy model. People become more assertive as they become more informed. They demand information, value for money, and are not so easily placated. Women in health and social care therefore need to grow into the skills demanded of them, develop their confidence, and become more assertive. The first step is to build self-esteem, belief in your own abilities, and reduce self-blame.

WORK BLOCKS FOR WOMEN

EXERCISE 2

Mark if the following raise any issues for you.

➤ **Honesty:** you are less guarded than you need to be. Revealing only what you want to reveal is not only necessary for self-protection, but also implies the ability to keep confidences.

➤ **Rules:** you take apparent rules literally. Men learn early in life that there are really two sets of rules – overt and covert.

➤ **Efficiency:** you think that efficiency is key. This might be the ideal, but in business work gets done through networking and an intricate set of relationships and office politics.

➤ **Niceness:** remember that you are liked or disliked on the basis of all your actions and your whole character.

➤ **Authority/awe:** you see yourself as weak, and those in authority as powerful. This prevents you from having the kind of productive team relationships with higher-level people that are essential to moving ahead.

➤ **Political:** the higher one goes in the workplace, the more one's success depends on being able to combine competence with political ability, a sense of strategy and human relations skills.

➤ **Socialisation:** you see the social side of work as wasting time, but it may well be an essential aspect of the job once you are in a more senior position.

➤ **Competition:** you feel inadequate, and steer away from competition for fear that you will lose. Or, conversely, you fear you will win, and thus humiliate your competitors. However, as you develop your skills and recognise the value of competition, you will fear failure less.

➤ **Female:** you feel compelled to play a 'feminine', naive role, and express shock and disbelief at some of the ways of the business world. This attitude does not win respect, but cuts you off from sources of information.

Research shows that while men look outside themselves to see why things have gone wrong, women look inside, and blame themselves.[2] Accepting fault feels more comfortable. It avoids conflict, nurtures others and smoothes over relationships. This can be challenged by acting in a positive, constructive way.

Combat some basic stereotyping by following some suggestions from Anne Dickson's *The Mirror Within*.[3]

---

2   Tannen D. *You Just Don't Understand: women and men in conversation*. Virago Press; 1992.

3   Dickson A. *The Mirror Within*. Quartet Books; 1985.

Stereotype A: Women are only interested in personal life

➤ Demonstrate your commitment. Women may be regarded as temporary members of the workforce until they prove otherwise. Talk to those above you about your plans and ambitions.

➤ On important occasions, arrive early and stay late. Make it clear that you do have an outside life – but you want to do what is needed because you are involved in your job.

➤ Let it be known that you carry your work home: 'I was reading an article last night on such-and-such that suggested a solution to …'

Stereotype B: Women need looking after

➤ Look like a woman who takes complete financial responsibility for herself. Your career is a permanent part of your life.

➤ Leave your personal life at home. If you have children, make your calls to the child-minder short, in break time, and do not discuss the situation with your colleagues. Put away the family photos.

➤ When personal problems get in the way of your work, demonstrate your reliability. Be seen as a self-sufficient adult who can handle responsibility and act on her own initiative.

➤ Do not just present problems: confront and solve them.

➤ Use the active voice. You are not asking permission. Instead of 'May I?' and 'Can I?', use 'I'm planning to' and 'I've decided to'.

➤ Do not appear to avoid adult responsibility by deferring to a 'parent': 'I have to ask my partner' or 'I don't know if they will let me'. Put yourself in an adult role by getting your own information, and be your own decision maker.

➤ Do not diminish yourself: use your full adult name at work – Deborah not Debs.

➤ Search out role models whom you particularly admire and learn what there is about their behaviour and appearance that could help enhance your image.

Stereotype C: Women need to toughen up

The big danger for a lot of women lies in seeming to be too malleable. Do not think you are making an assertion just by making a protest. In negotiations, people will push hard to get the best deal they can, so if you raise an issue, make it effectual. If you postpone the issue, you display weakness and compliance. Do not assume that if you are reasonable, your adversary will respond by also being reasonable. Be assertive.

> Asserter: 'We agreed on £3000; I simply won't pay more.'

Over-charger: 'You didn't tell us about all the difficulties with this particular system. We have lost hundreds of pounds.'

Asserter: 'I'm sorry you lost money, but the agreed price is £3000.'

Over-charger: 'You're being unreasonable. Everyone knows things have to be adjusted when there are problems.'

Asserter: 'I am sympathetic to your situation, but we did discuss our parameters, and a deal's a deal.'

In summary, we have seen that women are expected by society to be more compliant than challenging and more obedient than ambitious. Other qualities, like leadership, taking full responsibility for the outcome of things and risk-taking, are not encouraged. But these are the very things required of us in the world of work. Thus we have to work so much harder than men at being assertive in order to move forward and begin to take charge of our lives.

KEY POINTS

➤ There are gender-specific roles and expectations that play out in our society. Men and women differ in their life experience, in their presentation and socialisation. Different opportunities exist for each.

➤ Assertiveness is particularly important for women. In terms of assertiveness, we look at patriarchy and feminism to explain the sense of inferiority that women have. Personal, political and cultural approaches are needed to understand why we behave as we do.

➤ Woman are socialised to become highly sensitised to the needs of others. Our default setting is non-confrontational. Our compassion traps us.

➤ Men generally find it easier to be assertive, but some find it harder to develop the fine-tuned and complex verbal and non-verbal skills needed to listen and communicate with empathy, sympathy and focus.

➤ Language enables us to communicate in many different ways, for many different purposes. The way the sentence is phrased, the syntax – word order – will also have an impact. Gender and culture differences mean that things said one way are interpreted differently by others. There are differences in the way men and women vie for power, for status and connection in their communication styles.

➤ As women model good professional and management behaviour, we break down prejudices and help men to form new expectations of us.

➤ The health service is still a hierarchical organisation with unwritten rules at play. This is shifting: those in less powerful positions are gaining more confidence and authority to question the medical ascendancy model.

➤ Work blocks for women: we can be too honest, are too nice, we need to learn to develop a sense of strategy and see socialising as an important part of work. We need to begin to look like women who take complete responsibility for themselves.

➤ We need to recognise the value of competition, accept responsibility, challenge our accusers, convert blame into action, live by our own standards, and choose when to apologise. We may take on certain beliefs about ourselves because we feel powerless to reject them, but it is possible to reconsider and change them.

FURTHER READING

Back K, Back K. *Assertiveness at Work: a practical guide to handling awkward situations.* 3rd ed. McGraw-Hill Professional; 2005.

Jeffers S. *Feel The Fear and Do it Anyway: how to turn your fear and indecision into confidence and action.* 20th Anniversary ed. Vermilion; 2007.

Jeffers S. *The Little Book of Confidence.* Rider Books; 1999.

Speer SA. *Gender Talk. Feminism, discourse and conversation analysis.* Routledge; 2005.

Swiss D. *The Male Mind at Work: a woman's guide to working with men.* Basic Books; 2001.

CHAPTER 3

How to be assertive

To become assertive, one has to notice and overcome difficulties by identifying and changing dysfunctional thinking, behaviour and emotional responses. This will involve developing skills for modifying beliefs, identifying distorted thinking, relating to others in different ways and changing behaviours. You will need to gain awareness of and test your beliefs and assumptions about yourself and your world, and identify how some of your usually unquestioned thoughts and behaviours are distorted or dysfunctional, unrealistic or unhelpful. Once those thoughts have been challenged, your feelings and your behaviours have a chance to change. This chapter gives a summary of some of the skills you need to become more assertive: for those interested in the detail, *see* Section 2, Assertiveness in practice, in my sister book, *Developing Assertiveness Skills for Health and Social Care Professionals*, where you will be led through how to be assertive in specific situations, such as negotiating, dealing with criticism, anger and conflict, and unwanted requests.

HOW TO BE ASSERTIVE

Assertive communication is honest and direct; it is speaking your mind without fudging the issue or being aggressive. The assertive speaker is prepared to:
➤ be specific
➤ be honest and open
➤ negotiate
➤ repeat their message if misunderstood
➤ compromise, if it is reasonable to do so
➤ listen
➤ self-disclose – express their feelings
➤ innovate – take chances and risks
➤ accept criticism, where appropriate
➤ prompt others to express themselves honestly.

Assertive communication usually leaves both speaker and listener feeling more comfortable than avoidance or confrontational communication.

To develop personally and professionally, we also need to protect and take care of ourselves by setting personal boundaries, to be able to tell other people when they are acting in ways that are not acceptable to us. We also need to learn how to acknowledge and understand our own feelings, to 'own' our own voice, and the right to speak up for ourselves. It is impossible to have a good, healthy relationship with someone who has no boundaries, with someone who cannot communicate directly, and honestly.

Many working in the caring professions are already skilled communicators, as they are selected for, or trained in, interpersonal communication skills. However, we all have black spots, so it is worth reflecting on some of your own skills.

Step 1: Understand yourself

In order to recognise assertiveness in yourself, question whether there is a pattern in the way you interact with people, and remember the times when something you did or said worked well. It is likely that if the communication went well, one of you was being assertive.

Use the following exercises to begin to understand yourself, to find out how you are likely to respond in a given situation, with whom, and under which circumstances. If you are interested in understanding more about how and why you, or others, behave as they do in more detail, *see* Chapter 4, Understanding ourselves, in Section 2.

EXERCISE 1

Write a list of five situations in which you would like to behave more assertively, with open, direct and honest communication.

Then, next to each situation, note your current response:

P = passive, A= aggressive or I = indirect (manipulative)

What do you see as an alternative, assertive response?

EXERCISE 2

List *who*, in friendships, work or family, makes you feel either passive or aggressive.
List *when* you have behaved non-assertively.
List *what* makes you feel, and behave, non-assertively, for example, when making mistakes or expressing negative feelings.

Step 2: The basics of assertive behaviour

The basic skills of assertiveness are relatively easy to learn and begin to use daily in situations that are not too challenging, provocative or difficult, but they do need practice. The following teaches us useful ways of communicating in difficult or problematic situations – when dealing with critical comments or manipulative behaviour, when having to give criticism, or when negotiating. It is hard to change ingrained habits of behaviour, so the general rule is to pause and think before you speak, prepare/rehearse your speech with sympathetic friends or colleagues and remember that if the situation is problematic or awkward for, you are more likely to hesitate, digress, make mistakes. We can only learn from the mistakes, so have a go!

1   Be clear and specific
➤ Make the statement brief, and avoid unnecessary padding, especially when saying 'no' – 'sorry' and 'but' dilute the clarity and expose your uncertainty.
➤ Own your statement, assume responsibility.
➤ Keep your statement simple, brief and direct.
➤ If uncertain what is meant by a comment, ask for clarity and examples, to expose the criticism.

2   Be open and honest about your feelings
➤ Tell how you feel, own it.
➤ Do not hide behind words.
➤ Do not use words to manipulate or hurt.
➤ Never say: 'You make me feel …' No one can make us feel anything; we take personal responsibility for our own feelings.
➤ Begin difficult situations with simple statements: 'I feel nervous/guilty/ angry …'

As we are rarely given the opportunity to explore negative feelings, this skill takes practice. To begin with, you may wish to note the impact of your feelings physically, in your body, for example, a sinking feeling, a lump in the throat, a tight chest, sickness. Name these, and then eventually you will feel more able to respond honestly and quickly.

3   Repeat your message
This technique is sometimes called the 'stuck record' or 'broken record' technique. If you feel misunderstood, or need to diffuse anger, calmly repeat your statement or request. Through such gentle persistence, you can maintain your position without falling prey to manipulative comment, irrelevant logic or argumentative bait. This is an especially useful skill to use when dealing with aggressive people:
➤ listen carefully to the other person's point of view
➤ acknowledge it
➤ then stick to your desired point
➤ repeat several times if necessary.

This technique is best used in situations when your time and energy is precious, or when your rights are in danger of being abused, or if someone is drawing you into their own agenda with irrelevant 'baits' or logic. One of the most effective benefits of using repetition in this way is that once you have prepared what you are going to say, you can relax and stay with your prepared argument, without panicking that you will need to think on your feet: however manipulative or bullying the other person is, you know exactly what needs to be said. There may be a situation when both parties are being assertive, in which case neither will want to continue for long, so will work towards a compromise fairly quickly.

4 *Fielding the response*

This I consider one of the most fundamental of all assertive skills. In order successfully to 'field' or 'fog' a response, you need to be able to indicate that you have heard what the other person has said, without getting 'hooked' by what they say. Thus you are able to show that you respect the other person's point of view without necessarily sharing it. In order to communicate effectively, you need to listen and indicate that you have heard what is said, and acknowledge it, but stick to your guns. This skill is especially useful when handling direct or indirect criticism. Fogging, or fielding, the response in this way allows you to receive criticism comfortably without becoming anxious or defensive. It also gives no reward to those manipulating you through unjustified criticism – people who use criticism to diminish your self-esteem rather than in addressing the issue to help you to understand yourself better.

When fielding, you need to be emotionally intelligent, and be aware of all the verbal and non-verbal messages that are being communicated or leaking out. The other person needs to know that you understand their motives and feelings as well as their thoughts. Listen out for the underlying issues (e.g. is the person angry, frustrated or irritated?).

Having shown that you are listening sympathetically, you are then able to continue confidently with your statement or answer; you are demonstrating that you are trying to understand the other person's point of view, but still hold your own. You need not be drawn into an explanation unless you chose to.

5 *Negotiate*

➤ Be prepared to negotiate for what you want, as assertion does not mean always getting your own way!
➤ Co-operate, bargain as equals, work as a partnership towards achieving something you both want.
➤ Use tact and forethought.
➤ Empathise, co-operate, trade.
➤ Avoid confrontation.
➤ Seek the common ground.

➤ Aim for a win-win situation.
➤ Listen to the other party's point of view before you begin to bargain.
➤ Make certain that you fully understand the other person's position – ask for clarification if necessary.
➤ Prepare yourself well beforehand: harness the facts and figures that help you in supporting your case.
➤ Make certain that you keep to the point: if you feel the conversation is side tracking, bring the discussion back to the central issue – if necessary use the 'broken record' technique.

Effective negotiation should end with both parties agreeing to a situation they both feel happy about – neither one is compromised – but this does not always happen. Sometimes one party has to back down. This does not necessarily mean that you have 'lost' if you do not get what you want. Reward yourself for making a courageous effort.

6   Compromise

Compromise results when both parties have negotiated from an equal position. When moving towards a workable compromise, a solution is found that takes the needs of both parties into consideration.
➤ Do not wait for the other person to 'give in' first: offer a compromise.
➤ Bargain for material goods, but never compromise on your self-respect.
➤ If you feel your personal worth is being questioned, respond as if you are being criticised.
➤ Remain objective and impartial.
➤ You may need to give way to stubbornness: if so, acknowledge this.

There is no compromise about feelings: you have to respect another person's feelings as he or she does your own. Assertive behaviour is fair: there is no win/lose but a mutually successful outcome. To compromise is to concede, to meet half way. See if you can view compromise as making a virtue of necessity.

7   Accepting criticism

This skill helps you to handle constructive criticism from others, by agreeing with or accepting criticism if appropriate instead of reacting to it as if an accusation. Like self-disclosure, this allows you to look more comfortably at the less positive aspects of your own personality or behaviour without denying that that behaviour exists or becoming defensive. At the same time, it reduces your critic's hostility. Examples of your response may be as follows.

'Yes, I know I can be aggressive at times.'

'You are right, I am untidy.'

'That's fair enough, I can be indecisive. I'm working on ways to speed up.'

Only agree with the criticism if it is fair or truthful. If you acknowledge the probability of truth in the comment, it disarms the critic, and you demonstrate that you remain your own judge. If someone criticises you directly, learn to acknowledge and agree with the criticism, but only if you feel that the criticism is fair or truthful.

8   Expressing feelings

The importance of understanding and sharing feelings cannot be underestimated in any discussion on assertion.

➤ Learn to identify, or clarify, how you feel before responding to any situation.
➤ Learn to identify what your emotions are telling you.
➤ Talk about your feelings with another person.
➤ Share some of your vulnerability.

Personal exposure does carry a risk, but it is an important part of the openness and honesty of being assertive. There is more about working with feelings in Section 2, Assertiveness and leadership in the workplace.

9   Prompting others to express themselves

This skill allows you more comfortably to seek out criticism of yourself, while prompting the other person to express negative feelings with more honesty. It can improve communication, especially in close relationships, and also encourages your critics to be more assertive. For example, if you suspect that the person you are talking to is hiding her true (negative) feelings, you may ask:

'Are you finding me difficult to talk to?'

'Do you think I am being unfair?'

'Does it seem as though I am pushing you into a corner again?'

'I hear you saying that you think I am disorganised, is that right?'

When behaving assertively, you are confronting issues and situations rather than waiting passively in the hope that you will be able to respond. It is less stressful, and more powerful, to set the agenda yourself.

There are times in any conversation when we suspect that there is 'something going on' beneath the surface. Often it is an intuitive feeling, or a suspicion that something is being said 'between the lines'. At times like this, follow your intuition and take the initiative to seek out, or prompt, an honest response.

10   Listen

The assertive person listens carefully.

➤ Watch and listen to the actual statement, and also for an underlying message.

➤ Learn to 'read' behind the words, and also to watch non-verbal behaviour for 'leakage' or signs that all is not as it seems.

➤ Clarify or check that you have heard correctly – this is a good way of stalling for time before responding if you cannot identify how you feel about a situation:

> 'So you think that I ought to be clearer about the facts?'

> 'Can I just check what you just said? ...'

Active listening is a physically demanding, conscious process of attending to what the speaker is saying. It requires the receiver to listen for the total meaning a person conveys, to try to determine both the content of the message and the feelings underlining it. Active listeners note all the cues, both verbal and non-verbal, in communication. When having a conversation with someone, try to spend more time listening than speaking. Let go of those initial urges to speak, and listen more. Listening can take tremendous effort, but, each time, you train your brain to become slightly more patient.[1]

Good listeners:

➤ listen: pay close, interested, attention

➤ paraphrase: demonstrate they have correctly perceived the sender's inner state and understood – 'Are you saying you dislike that kind of work ...?'

➤ ask questions to clarify the position, or reflect back that they have heard, for example, 'So that made you feel very angry?'

➤ never interrupt

➤ never advise or suggest solutions.

➤ allow feelings – they do not try not to stop them but encourage them; suppressing feelings will only increase the sender's discomfort and discourage them from trusting you.

11   Innovate

➤ Take charge and regain control.

➤ Act as your own catalyst for change.

➤ Innovate, and do not wait for others, or fate, to take over.

---

1   Alidina S. *Mindfulness for Dummies.* John Wiley & Sons; 2010. p. 53

Some people find that once they are able to let themselves set the scene for change in this way, other areas of their life are affected: they have the confidence to move ahead and perhaps alter the balance of control in their personal as well as professional life. Once you allow yourself to be assertive, you are acknowledging that you are no longer the passive victim of other people's manipulation. You are able to make your own decisions, and this can be a very powerful motivator for change.

12 Empower with compassion

Assertiveness is a very powerful and freeing tool. When we behave assertively, we experience very positive feelings, and those feelings inevitably become more meaningful, or central, to our lives. Assertive behaviour gives us a certain strength and stability; it allows us to have more influence and authority. This extra power is very energetic and potent, but must be used wisely. It is very tempting after years of feeling oppressed or restricted to rush out and regain the world! Allow room for negotiation or compromise.

Compassion and caring support each other: compassion brings caring to assertion, while assertion helps you feel comfortable giving compassion. Being empathetic can give you a lot of useful information about your communication partner – what is really on their mind, what they really care about. In seeing the bigger picture, you reduce any frustration or anger towards them. Any natural capacity for empathy can be strengthened by:

➤ setting the stage: orient yourself to the situation to come
➤ staying 'open' and tuned in to the other person
➤ noticing their actions, the non-verbal communication
➤ tuning into their expressions and feelings
➤ tracking their thoughts – what might he be feeling here? What could be most important to him? What might he want from me?[2]

In order to communicate compassionately and effectively, you will need to be mindful of, and stay in touch with, deeper feelings and desires. Keep asking yourself what you want/need. You will need to take personal responsibility for getting your needs met in relationships – it will help to:

➤ take turns to focus on each other's topics when talking, rather than mixing them together
➤ never try communicate with the aim to fix, change or convince another person – you can only take responsibility for yourself and your own feelings

---

2 Hanson R, Mendius R. *Buddha's Brain: the practical neuroscience of happiness, love and wisdom.* New Harbinger Publications; 2009. pp. 137–8.

➤ keep coming back to your own experience – emotions, underlying hopes and wishes – rather than the other person's actions and your opinions about them

➤ preface conversations with 'I feel ...', so that you 'own' your own feelings and actions

➤ stay guided by your own personal, moral code – avoid language that is fault-finding or inflammatory

➤ focus clearly on the present and future during the conversation, not the past

➤ give yourself time – remember that whatever is happening is impermanent; consider whether you will feel as charged about this in 10 years' time.

Once you have developed a stronger and more empathic communication style, you will find that over time, truths about other people become apparent. Does this person respect your boundaries? Keep agreements and promises? Repair misunderstandings? If not, consider minimising contact.[3] For example, you cannot make a co-worker stop being rude to you, but you can 'shrink' the relationship by minimising your contact with them.

Assertiveness helps you to stick up for yourself and others, and to feel confident that you can still get your needs met even while being compassionate. Be guided by virtue and principle, which regulate more healthy aims. If you stay bound by the key principles of being open to people, non-judgmental, staying connected and alert to possibility, you will be able to communicate more peacefully, with clarity, insight and understanding. When we behave assertively, it allows us to have more influence and authority within our professional role, and as human beings. In learning to be assertive, you are releasing untapped potential, and beginning a process of self-discovery through which you can begin to understand yourself, and others, more. Through being assertive you also empower others, allowing them the room to take space and negotiate their needs. As your sensitivity to others increases, so will your ability to feel care and compassion.

Use these skills wisely, and recognise that the learning process is slow. Assertiveness is something that takes many, many years to effect: after all, you are learning to undo several years' worth of habitually different behaviour. So go slowly, and accept that in learning to be assertive you are beginning a process of self-discovery through which you can begin to understand your true potential.

---

3   Hanson, Mendius, note 2 above, p. 152.

KEY POINTS

➤ In learning how to become assertive, habitual ways of communicating will be changed, and this needs courage, determination and practice.

➤ The work is based on testing beliefs and assumptions, and identifying how some of our usually unquestioned thoughts are distorted, unrealistic and unhelpful.

➤ The entirety of our adult life is spent making personal decisions and choices. If we accept this, we are free and empowered to accept any consequences of our decisions.

➤ We need to protect and take care of ourselves by setting personal boundaries – we need to be able to tell other people when they are acting in ways that are not acceptable to us.

➤ We need to acknowledge and understand our own feelings, to 'own' our own voice, and the right to speak up for ourselves.

➤ Assertiveness is a very powerful and freeing tool. When we behave assertively, we experience very positive feelings, and those feelings inevitably become more meaningful or central to our lives. This extra power is very energetic and potent, but must be used wisely.

➤ Compassion brings caring to assertion, while assertion helps us to feel comfortable giving compassion.

➤ In order to communicate compassionately and effectively, you will need to be mindful of, and stay in touch with, deeper feelings and desires. Keep coming back to your own experience rather than the other person's actions, and you will be 'owning' your own feelings and actions.

➤ Stay guided by your own personal, moral code.

➤ You will find that over time, truths about other people become apparent. Does this person respect your boundaries? Keep agreements and promises? Repair misunderstandings? If not, consider minimising contact.

➤ If you stay bound by the key principles of being open to people, non-judgmental, staying connected, alert and awake to possibility, you will be able to communicate more peacefully, with clarity, insight and understanding.

➤ Through being assertive, you also empower others, allowing them the room to take space and negotiate their needs.

➤ The assertive speaker is prepared to:
  - be clear and specific
  - be honest and open about their feelings
  - negotiate
  - repeat their message if misunderstood
  - compromise, if it is reasonable to do so
  - listen, 'field' or 'fog'
  - self-disclose: express their feelings

– innovate: take chances and risks
– accept criticism, where appropriate
– prompt others to express themselves honestly
– innovate, empower.

FURTHER READING

Beck K, Beck K. *Assertiveness at Work: a practical guide to handling awkward situations.* 3rd ed. McGraw-Hill Professional; 2005.

Bishop S. *Develop Your Assertiveness.* 2nd ed. Kogan Page; 2006.

Hadfield S, Hasson G. *How to be Assertive in Any Situation.* Pearson Prentice Hall Life; 2010.

Lindenfield G. *Assert Yourself: simple steps to getting what you want.* Thorsons; 2001.

Potts S. *Entitled to Respect: how to be confident and assertive in the workplace.* How To Books Ltd; 2010.

Smith MJ. *When I Say No I Feel Guilty.* Bantam USA; 1975.

Section 2

Assertiveness and leadership in the workplace

CHAPTER 4

Understanding ourselves

A BROAD LOOK AT COMMUNICATION

What are communication skills and why is it important for developing professionals to learn about them? We know that communication skills involve a whole raft of verbal and non-verbal skills: words (written or spoken), gestures and body language, delivery (tone of voice, pitch, timing), use of symbols (pictorial, numerical, etc.) and listening. Understanding how communication works is important as the ability to communicate well is directly related to our ability to be successful in life – our happiness, relationships, personal and professional growth all depend on effective communication. Good, if not excellent, communication is especially important for those in leadership positions as it assists them to make discoveries about themselves and others, solve problems and develop new skills, manage conflict, emotion and anger, understand other people and how they communicate and, most important, to manage themselves: to question their position, adapt, change and grow.

Others appreciate the listening ability, clarity and honesty of good communicators. Communication is a two-way process that involves sharing information. It is essential for getting along with others and getting things done.

This section aims to take health and social care workers, clinicians and managers, through all of these functions. We look underneath the surface levels of assertive communication, to see what underpins it. This chapter looks at how to improve and enhance our interpersonal communication skills so that we become more effective listeners, responding skilfully and sensitively to the challenges modern healthcare presents us with. The aim is that, through reading this book, you will change your ideas: changing ideas influences behaviour; and changing behaviour leads to changes in ideas. Many psychologists and cognitive behavioural therapists have cited these behavioural approaches as crucial in change management.[1]

---

1   Grieger R, Boyd J. *Rational-Emotive Therapy: a skills based approach.* Van Nostrand Reinhold; 1980. p. 187. Ellis A. *RETR and Assertiveness Training* [audiocassette]. Albert Ellis Institute for Rational-Emotive Behaviour Therapy; 1979. Beck AT, Rush AJ, Shaw BF, *et al. Cognitive Therapy of Depression.* The Guilford Press; 1979.

We have seen that most complaints arising in organisations are based around poor communication. To avoid this, both clinicians and those holding leadership responsibilities need to be multi-skilled. To be an effective team leader, you need to share ideas, concerns, suggestions and other information with those on your team, your superiors and people outside your organisation. As well as communicating with patients and clients, you may need to give work assignments or instructions, make or discuss changes in procedures, motivate or supervise, or solicit ideas, thoughts or information. The interpersonal communication skills needed for this are wide-based, functional or process-orientated, and include such tasks as motivating, leading, listening, instructing, organising; writing, presenting, chairing, counselling; facilitating; supervising, delegating, interviewing, appraising.

Each process has its own skill, and each skill can be learnt. Communication is complex. It involves:

➤ a message – statements, questions, commands or warnings
➤ a language – words, symbols and gestures make up the elements of language
➤ a system – communication occurs through touch, silence, voice, gestures, writing.

We know, for example, that language is important, but it is only one vehicle for communicating something. Language does have many useful functions, enabling us, among other things, to volunteer information, to respond, to state needs/likes/dislikes, to express feelings, to request, negotiate, direct, speculate, imagine, plan, organise, give an account or sequence, and to refer to past/future events. However, it is the way something is communicated – its delivery – that tells us more about the content. Facial expressions, smiles and frowns play a part in communication, as does:

➤ timing and speed – communication is affected when people talk too quickly, cut one another off or wait too long to bring up an issue
➤ body language – clenched fists, eye contact, head position
➤ word choice – will tell us if the situation is, public or private, doubtful or hopeful, formal or informal, serious or relaxed
➤ tone of voice – feelings such as sorrow or pride, anger, impatience, can all be expressed
➤ proximics – how people use and perceive the physical space around them.

Because communication is 7% verbal, and 93% non-verbal,[2] the language element is perhaps not as crucial as we once thought. And it is this that interests

---

2 Mehrabian A, Ferris S. Inference of attitudes from nonverbal communication in two channels. *Journal of Consulting Psychology*. 1967; **31**(3): 248–52.

us. We have to make big efforts to communicate: words and symbols have different meanings among different cultures. Humour may help or hinder; gestures can be misinterpreted. We can never assume our communication is understood or accepted by others: good communicators always check that they have been understood.

WHY IS COMMUNICATION SO IMPORTANT?

It was Argyle[3] who first postulated that whereas spoken language is normally used for communicating information about events external to the speakers, non-verbal codes are used to establish and maintain interpersonal relationships. Many of those working in healthcare have lost sight of the importance of communication – there is so much to do and so little time to accomplish what is needed. When stretched, it seems quicker and easier to get on with a job, and keeping people informed feels difficult because there is so much to do and tell.

Those leading need to make a commitment to employee communication. Not to inform is to patronise – if we assume the staff do not need to know, they will feel undervalued and disrespected. Communication has to be two way – all employees have views, good ideas or suggestions on alternatives ways of working; leaders ask and are prepared to listen. Other people often have a clear outside vision on a project, whereas those working daily on the practicalities and details may lose sight of its simplicity. Managers and the most qualified do not always have the answers. Of course, if we accept that visibility and openness is important, we need to recognise that mistakes will be aired in the same way as the triumphs.

THE PROCESS OF COMMUNICATION

Consider some of functions of communication in more detail.

Communication is multi-directional – it can be impersonal, often written, directional, and one way:

➤ it can be face to face
➤ it can be outward – towards the public or government, for example
➤ it can also go 'up' from employees to employer
➤ it can go sideways – if you utilise team work.

To communicate successfully, people need skills which can be learned or applied. Different types of meeting, for example, have different functions. Each one may utilise a different set of skills – chairing, facilitating, presenting,

---

3 Argyle M, Salter V, Nicholson H, *et al.* The communication of inferior and superior attitudes by verbal and non-verbal signals. *British Journal of Social and Clinical Psychology.* 1970; **9**: 222–31.

team building, instructing, etc. If communication is defined as the exchange of information between a sender and receiver with the inference of meaning, an individual's personality, history, motivation and personal development all affect the way she or he hears, or receives, information transmitted by another. These all affect communication accuracy. Some other less visible factors also have a big influence: the organisational structure, the interpersonal power imbalances within and, of course, incomplete information.

The organisational structure

Communication is a central organisational process. The exchange of information between different participants links the various subsystems of the organisation, and build and reinforce interdependence between them.

The NHS works within strictly hierarchical lines, with superiors (the medics/managers) and subordinates (the staff). This arrangement can create communication difficulties, with the lower-status members – those without much power – suppressing unfavourable information because they worry that their superiors may regard them unfavourably if they pass on negative material. Thus, less powerful members only communicate what they feel you want to hear. Depending where you fit into this hierarchy, you may or may not be party to these negative comments. If you are a practice manager who considers the partners your peers, you will feel happier passing on 'bad' news to them. However, you then may not hear all you need to from your subordinates. On the other hand, if you stand with the staff, and represent their voice, you may find it difficult to stand your ground with the doctors. A skilled communicator will fit somewhere between, and gain respect from both.

The larger and more specialised that the work groups are within your organisation, the greater the possibility for misunderstanding, as the employees in different teams have access to a different amount of, and very different, information. This discourages sharing and increases the potential for misunderstandings. Differences in power, goals and expertise between departments (finance, personnel or secretarial, reception, management, nursing) may make communication difficult and allow discord, gossip and backbiting to flourish.

Interpersonal relationships

The relationship between the two people communicating also affects the accuracy with which messages are given and received. An important factor in this is how much *trust* there is between the two: when people trust each other, communication tends to be more accurate and open. When the receiver of the message has considerable *influence* over the sender, the communication may be modified or guarded – it would make sense that someone seeking promotion would modify their message in a way that enhances their position or personal development. *Group norms*, or expected standards of behaviour, may limit the amount or type of information people feel they can legitimately discuss. The type and content of communication differs in different contexts too – the relaxed chat of the staff room differs from the more formal discussion in meetings.

Incomplete information

This is particularly relevant when an employee's performance is being appraised or discussed. If relying on only one source of information when judging performance, persistent biases are likely to occur.

So, what are some of the barriers to effective communication and how can we make ourselves heard above these?

BARRIERS TO EFFECTIVE COMMUNICATION

Lack of feedback

If we communicate something without any acknowledgement that we have been heard and understood, we cannot assume that our message has been understood. Managers often give large quantities of information and direction without provision or opportunity for their staff to indicate that they have understood. There are various reasons why this happens, such as lack of trust in the other's ability to contribute, lack of personal confidence ('They might think I don't know the answer'), an assumption that people have the same goals, ideals and motivations as ourselves ('But it's obvious I meant …'), or even poor communication skills – where two-way communication is not respected.

Everyone has a responsibility to encourage two-way communication. If staff fail to inform their bosses about their needs and values, or withhold information because they distrust their bosses or are antagonistic, bosses have a responsibility to redefine the trust. Communication should be as open as possible, and one way that can be made possible is to create a supportive communication climate where people feel able to talk without feeling judged.

Clearly, good managers *avoid* the following behaviours.

➤ **Ridicule, lecturing**, being dismissive, ordering. *Instead*, communicate respectfully.
➤ **Evaluating:** when we behave defensively we judge – we blame, call for different behaviour, praise. *Instead*, create a supportive environment by giving and asking for information – behave more neutrally.
➤ **Controlling:** when we attempt to persuade others by imposing our personal attitudes on them. *Instead*, collaborate with your colleague by defining and solving the problem together.
➤ **Strategic communication:** when we attempt to manipulate others, *instead* of dealing more spontaneously, openly and without deception.

➤ **Uncaring behaviour:** *instead*, demonstrate your concern; show empathy by identifying with your colleagues position.

➤ **Superiority:** *instead*, show your respect for others by de-emphasising the status and power differences.

➤ **Certainty:** being dogmatic, wanting to win rather than solve the problem. *Instead*, show your openness to new information and interpretations; postpone taking sides.

Noise

Interference that occurs during the communication process is called noise; it may be audible or inaudible. The presence of a silent third party during a conversation may act as noise in that it distracts the receiver from hearing what the speaker says. The receiver's preoccupation with an unrelated problem can have the same effect.

The use of language

The choice of words or language in which a sender encodes a message will influence the quality of communication. Because language is an abstract representation of a phenomenon, there is room for interpretation and distortion of the meaning. Misunderstandings can arise through using words that are too abstract, too general or too vague. Jargon and technical terms frequently create misunderstanding, as does the use of slang or colloquialisms.

Language enables us to communicate in many different ways, for many different purposes. We do not always mean what we say.[4]

We can speak the same word or sentence with altogether different meanings, with the meaning conveyed in the tone (of voice), the stress, pausing, intonation or context. The way the sentence is phrased, the syntax – word order – will also have an impact.

Argyle[5] was one of the first psychologists to put forward the hypothesis that whereas spoken language is normally used for communicating information about events external to the speakers, non-verbal codes are used to establish and maintain interpersonal relationships. Paralinguistics is the term used for the study of how things are said and how this affects the meaning of what is said. It looks at language purposes, some of the hidden meanings, expectations and assumptions in our language, some of the ways we communicate, and includes the study of how men and women's discourse differs.

---

4   Townsend J. Paralinguistics: it's not what you say it's the way that you say it. *Management Decision*. 1988; **26**(3): 26–40. Crystal D. Prosody and paralinguistic correlates of social categories. In: Gardener E, editor. *Social Anthropology and Language*. Tavistock; 1971. pp. 185–206.

5   Argyle, Salter, Nicholson, *et al.*, note 3 above.

There are always hidden meanings beneath language. It has an unstated but 'heard' hierarchical ranking/power dynamic that plays out. Rank is insidious and crucial. Compliments are almost always given by those of higher rank to those of lower rank, and talk/subject matter is always initiated by the higher ranking. This ranking means that unspoken rules are followed: there are hidden expectations and assumptions in the meaning behind the language. Thus, if a person of higher 'rank' asks 'You don't mind if I do X do you?', there is an expectation that the person of lower rank will accede.

Both genders have different repertoires, and we have different expectations about how men and women present, their expectations, their core beliefs. This affects the way people – the public, our patients/clients, managers – view us, so it is important to acknowledge. Deborah Tannen[6] is one of the biggest researchers into language discourse and gender. She demonstrates how, for example, men and women, girls and boys, differ in their use of 'air time', the type of vocabulary used, levels of directness, how they use silence versus volubility to indicate status or connection. Her work shows how women tend towards connection and sharing, men towards hierarchy, problem solving and building status. Men often have the confidence to interrupt, but are more likely to interrupt someone of lower rank, women included. They are more likely to use expressions of conflict and verbal aggression, raise topics of interest to themselves and behave with high confidence. Women have some known conversational rituals, with more frequent apology. Thus there is a hidden agenda in any discourse, where conversation plays out hidden issues of patriarchy, power and solidarity.

Listening deficiencies

The quality of the receiver's listening may help or hurt communication. Effective communication calls for active listening by individuals. Assertive people have fine-tuned their listening and hearing skills. Active listening requires the receiver to listen for the total meaning a person conveys; to try to determine both the content of the message and the feelings underlining it. Active listening also calls for noting all the cues, both verbal and non-verbal, in communication. A good listener understands, shows awareness (eye contact, interprets facial expression and body language), reflects back, takes turns, does not interrupt, initiates when appropriate, questions appropriately, gets to your level (literally), and attempts to tune in, to 'speak your language'.

---

6 Tannen D. *You Just Don't Understand: women and men in conversation*. Virago; 1992. Tannen D. *Talking From 9 to 5: women and men at work: language, sex and power*. Virago; 1996.

IMPROVE YOUR ABILITY TO BE HEARD

Healthy organisations seem to be strongly influenced by humanistic psychology, where openness, trust and belief in individual growth are paramount, and build an organisational framework that is humanitarian, where the management style is open, reflective, listening and interested. For this to happen, be prepared to learn how to communicate well.

How do you communicate verbally at work?
Through writing – emails, reports, team meetings? The phone? Note down why you think there may be crossed wires in each situation.

In any communication, both sides need to:
➤ be interested and involved
➤ be willing to be open and honest
➤ feel heard and understood.

➤ The atmosphere must be comfortable.
➤ Even if the talking is difficult, the important things get said.

Conversations have to make a difference. Something useful or satisfying happens as a result.

Make a note of the good and poor communicators in your team.

Good communication	Poor communication
Working together in partnership	Scoring points to win
Co-operative, nurturing	Competitive
Makes feelings clear	Hides feelings, defensive
Explains their needs	Applies pressure, bullies
Shares the airtime	Dominates the airtime
Responds sensitively	Insensitive behaviour
Understands that everyone has a different inner world, and different motivations and experiences	Wants everyone to be like themselves, makes assumptions
Understands why the conversation is taking place	Misunderstands
Is open to whatever	Attacks or threatens
Is interested by difference	Patronises or puts down
Listens and watches	Ignores
Advises and supports	Lectures, critical, judgemental

Good communication	Poor communication
Knows themselves, and is true to self	Constructs a false public persona
Values your experience	Gives unwanted advice, preaches
Listens	Does not pay attention
Respects and values your views	Trivialises views
Clarity, stays on track	Rambles
Reflects back to show understanding, responds with interest	Always misses the point
Welcomes difficulties and conflict as opportunities to learn	Avoids conflict
Checks out it is a good time to talk	Barges in regardless
Is open minded	Is closed minded
Balances questions with talking about self	Asks too many questions, interrogates
Allows plenty of time	Impatient
Cut the tale up into bite-size chunks	Dumps too much information
Gives people the opportunity to respond	Overloads or bores
Encourages the flow	Avoids
Prompts	Takes up all the room
Asks	Tells

Effective communication
➤ Devote the time.
➤ Share.
➤ Keep in regular contact.
➤ Be assertive.
➤ Be specific.
➤ Be clear.
➤ Be open.
➤ Be prepared to negotiate.
➤ Value difference.
➤ Own your own thoughts and feelings. Use 'I' instead of 'you'; describe your feelings instead of the other person's behaviour: ' I feel angry because I don't like having to start all over again' instead of 'I feel angry when you are late'.
➤ Respect and recognise feelings.
➤ Do not assume.
➤ Repeat the message if misunderstood.
➤ Compromise if it is reasonable to do so.
➤ Listen to the other person.
➤ Accept responsibility.
➤ Choose the right moment.
➤ Summarise.
➤ Keep an open mind.

➤ Show you understand, and say when you do not.
➤ Do not give advice unless asked for it.
➤ Base any feedback on facts.
➤ Sandwich a negative between two positives.
➤ Express your feelings.
➤ Innovate – take chances and risks.
➤ Accept criticism, when appropriate.
➤ Prompt others to express themselves honestly.
➤ Empower yourself.
➤ Be yourself.

In summary, good communicators:

➤ read the situation	➤ look for clues
➤ engage attention	➤ check understanding
➤ make the meaning clear	➤ say what is on their mind
➤ tell the story	➤ summarise.

Non-verbal communication

How you dress, the apparent wealth and status reflected in your surroundings, and your time and space could clarify the meaning of verbal communication or increase its impact. Non-verbal signals may also contradict a verbal message or alter its meaning. In manager/subordinate communication there are also the obstacles to frank expressions of opinion or full disclosure of information. A good communicator watches out for the signs of contradiction or discomfort and encourages a more honest discourse. If you indicate your authority non-verbally through power-dressing or use of office space, you may need to make more effort to meet others more equally. Watch for the non-verbal signs of dominance around your workplace.
➤ Who holds the biggest space, the largest consulting room?
➤ A clear, uncluttered desk and surroundings?

The higher up the organisation you go, the less you have to *do* (dirty your hands) – your job is just to think. An insecure manager may place their desk a considerable distance from the door, so whoever comes in has to walk a distance before being within communicable distance – a very exposing and humbling experience. Unless you need to remind your staff you mean business, create a more comfortable, less oppressive communication environment and sit them at right angles not opposite you, without placing a desk between you. Status should come to you through being respected, not feared.

Watch out to see whether the non-verbal messages you are receiving or giving serve to underline or undermine the verbal message. If the latter, try creating a more supportive communication climate in order to get and give a clearer picture.

Listen actively[7]

Without confusing the professional role of counsellor in the practice, most of us at times need to adopt a first line counselling role within our workplace. If anyone is distressed, angry or has something of import to say, your role is to listen.

➤ **Listen:** pay close, interested, attention.
➤ **Paraphrase:** demonstrate you have correctly perceived the sender's inner state and understood – 'Are you saying you dislike that kind of work …?
➤ **Ask questions:** to clarify the position or to reflect back that you have heard, for example, 'So that made you feel very angry?'.
➤ **Never interrupt**.
➤ **Never advise** or suggest solutions.
➤ **Allow feelings:** do not try not to stop them, but encourage them – suppressing feelings will only increase the sender's discomfort and discourage them from trusting you.

If people have the chance to talk, uninterrupted and with your full attention, they unravel the problem themselves.

Avoid discriminating language

Take care around the use of offensive language, and challenge it if you hear it. Unwitting prejudice, ignorance, thoughtlessness and stereotyping do nothing but disadvantage those in the minority. This prejudice often extends to discriminate against sexuality, class, disability or culture as well as race.

Certain factors in our society will shift our sense of power in relation to others.[8]

Factors which shift power up	Factors which shift the power down
Aged between 25 and 45	Young or old
Middle or upper class	Working class
White	Black or from an ethnic minority
English speaking	A strong regional accent
Articulate	Not speaking English well, stammering

---

7 Bailey A. *Talk Works: British Communications plc*. BT education material. Available at: www.btplc. com/Responsiblebusiness/Supportingourcommunities/Learningandskills/Freeresources/ AllTalk/Default.aspx (accessed May 2013).
8 Sourced from: Cruse Bereavement Care. *Making it Happen: working towards equality in Cruse Bereavement Care*. Available at: www.crusebereavementcare.org.uk (accessed April 2013).

Factors which shift power up	Factors which shift the power down
Educated	Uneducated
Employed	Unemployed
Able bodied	Disabled in any way
Tall	Short
Attractive	Perceived as 'ugly'
Male	Female
Professional	Unemployed
Rich	Poor
Average	Different in any way, for example, through culture, sexuality, having an obvious mental health problem or a victim (of violence, abuse)

How can you avoid offending and patronising others?

➤ What are your feelings about the above?

➤ What assumptions and attitudes do you already hold?

➤ Why?

➤ How might these attitudes impact on other individuals around you?

➤ However you identify, think about the experience of your opposite number: what would it feel like to be more/less powerful?

➤ How do you act and behave when faced with your prejudice? Are you dismissive, patronising, hurtful, scared?

➤ Have you ever used a term that would upset or offend?

➤ Do you make assumptions about people, for example, assume everyone is heterosexual?

➤ Have you ever been challenged about your use of language?

➤ Have you ever responded to the public in a way that could have deterred or inhibited them from using your services?

Have you ever examined some of your beliefs and prejudices about your patients, your colleagues? Human beings tend to act tribally: we feel safer in groups, and one way we reinforce this feeling of safety is to poke fun at or invalidate the 'other'. Fundamentally, we act through fear and ignorance. Think of all the negative ways certain groups of people can be described. Take care with your own language, and be prepared to challenge others if they use stereotypical, offensive descriptions ('bed blocker' for 'older person'; 'chairman' for 'chair'). Be aware that the preferred terms are fluid and changing, and some terms may be 'reclaimed' by minority groups themselves. Keep yourself familiar with current usage. What does offensive language tell us about our beliefs? Think about where these attitudes and beliefs have come from. Challenge yourself; question those beliefs. If we consider prejudices we may hold about migrants, for example, think about what would it take for you to leave your family, friends and culture and go to a place where you knew no one? What qualities do you think you would need to do this? List them.

Janet Suzman, actor and civil liberties campaigner, has said that dealing with racism is about having the courage not to let it go unchallenged. Racism lurks just below the surface in so many of us. If we feel that we have the permission to say ridiculous things, somebody with a conscience needs to stand up to us – or we to them.

Lateral communication

Once you have perfected the art of communicating upwards and downwards, you can then move on to tackling broader communication problems in general practice such as team building, leadership and motivating staff. The next section explores the wider processes of communication across the practice.

TIPS FOR EMERGING MANAGERS: IMPROVING COMMUNICATION

Those aspiring to leadership positions should be aware of some of the common communication pitfalls, and the ways to remediate them. The factors most commonly affecting complaints and clinical negligence claims within the NHS are: communication breakdowns, shown in either poor systems and processes or human error.[9] Because of this, we develop systems to manage clinical and administrative communications, for example, protocols, tracer systems, complaints procedures. Systems need to be put in place to integrate quality communication into all organisational processes. The basic considerations to avoid communication breakdown across people or systems are to plan ahead, problem solve, communicate (keep people involved and informed), and review and monitor.

Review any systems of communication across your team

Do you:
➤ create systems to identity and evaluate mistakes
➤ share good practice
➤ hold regular team meetings
➤ have clear policies, protocols, agreements
➤ implement and adhere to formal systems
➤ educate and feedback to staff?

Staff should be informed and consulted about matters likely to affect their employment. Those with a management role in the practice need to create a climate where equity for all and respect for individual differences are ensured.

---

9 Wilson J. General practice risk management. *News for Fundholders*. 1995; **12**: 4.

Communication rights should extend across the practice so that staff feel fully and properly trained to do the job they are employed to do, and able to comment or complain to their employers without fear or prejudice.

In keeping staff informed, consider whether your communication is one way only (an email, a notice).There are distinct advantages to this – everyone receives the same information, it is clear and unlikely to be misunderstood, it is relatively cheap. The disadvantage is that the communication is one way – so advise people where they can go if they want further information. Investigate more innovative ways of communicating (e.g. using social media to publicise your work), and keep them current.

It is courteous and necessary to devise procedures for keeping everyone in the team informed about how the team works – especially visiting clinicians and attached staff, who will need a current information pack or an induction manual. Incoming staff feel disorientated and uneasy when they have not got the information they need to hand, and the team resents having to stop work to give out information regularly.

A planned induction gives general and detailed information on the workings of the organisation. It should include:

➤ staff facilities, key codes, etc.
➤ procedures and protocols
➤ staff names, main responsibilities and timetables
➤ when and where the meetings are held
➤ who to contact if assistance is needed
➤ a list of needed local contact details, for example, hospital, pharmacy, social services, schools, clinics.

Arrange for the inductee to spend time with the essential staff. Allow time for them to become familiar with the appointments and visits book, appointing procedures, duty rota and telephone system. It is also very valuable for them to spend some time in the waiting room, to understand the public experience.

Demonstrate good communication habits

The Transmission Model of Communication[10]

| Encoding | | Sender | | Method | | Receiver | | Decoding |

The best leaders ask rather than command, and tell why it is important to know. They are positive – stress 'what to do' not 'what to avoid'. Requests should leave as much freedom of action as is possible to the receiver, con-

---

10 Fred Pryor Seminars. *How to Supervise People*. Pryor Resources, Inc.; 1997.

sistent with their ability and training. Always obtain feedback – add 'checking' to the above model. Do not assume that the person has got the message: Ask open-ended questions: 'What do you think?', not 'Is that clear?'. Take the initiative and assume ownership of potential misunderstandings: 'Sometimes I'm not sure I've made myself clear – would you run it back by me so I can check myself?' Watch for non-verbal signs of doubt or insecurity. Encourage and reward, never punish.

Tell them.
Show them.
Have them tell you.
Have them show you.
Have them write it down.

Teach good communication habits

Despite rapid increases in technology, paperwork is increasing. The way paperwork is processed directly affects how smoothly an organisation runs. To communicate well in business can bring positive results. Assertive managers do not fudge: to limit losses and avoid breakdowns in communication, make explicit your expected standards.

Communicating with your public

Literature

Keeping people informed improves communication, assists in managing risk and supports clinical governance guidelines. This section looks some of the best ways to keep patients and clients informed about the services you offer. The information may be in the form of a newsletter or leaflets or provided on a website. However it is presented, it must be updated regularly and written in language appropriate for your target audience, given that the average reading age in this country is equivalent to an educated nine-year-old: the level of a tabloid newspaper. Recently a scientist at the University of Bath looked at pages about diabetes on 15 internet health sites run mainly by charities and official bodies.[11] He found people would need a reading ability of an educated 11- to 17-year-old to understand the sites. The researcher found the NHS Direct online site used the most complicated language and was the hardest to understand, with people needing the reading ability of an educated person aged 16 to comprehend information. To avoid this:

---

11 Boulos M. Analysing www.diabetes-help.com. University of Bath; 2004.

Use plain English

➤ translate if required

➤ use words of one to two syllables

➤ keep all sentences and paragraphs short

➤ keep language personal: 'You, we, your baby' instead of 'They, those'

➤ avoid polysyllabic words/double-negatives/jargon/acronyms

➤ the aim is to inform not to impress – be specific not vague

➤ repeat key information several times

➤ use positive language

➤ plan and test with those you are writing for

➤ use a large font, and print black on yellow to make it accessible to those with visual impairments.

Instead of	Try
Our aim for this leaflet is to	We aim to
Keep you up to date with all of our services	Tell you about our: ➤ doctors ➤ nurses ➤ health visitors ➤ counsellor
We hope patients will find this information useful when deciding whether to see a doctor – or whether someone else in our team can help you	Point you in the right direction
It is not yet possible to	We are trying to

MEETINGS

Best practice shows us organisations where the decision making is devolved down and ideas are fed up. Teams that make good use of meeting time go a long way towards alleviating those problems. If meetings are private, develop a mechanism to feed back to the staff following private meetings and external reviews. Staff need to feel included in the major decision making. Here are some facts about meetings in general:

➤ most people do not like meetings

➤ meetings are essential to foster good two-way communication

➤ meetings need to be held regularly

➤ employers demonstrate their commitment to their employees through attending meetings

➤ staff need to feel included in the major decision making.

Note whether your meetings are well chaired, organised, well attended, held frequently enough, include agendas and minutes. Begin to unpick/analyse some of the difficulties. Challenge problems, do not bury them.

How often are meetings held?	Are they managed well?	What are the problems?
Diary meetings		
Informal open meetings		
Whole team meetings		
Partnership meetings		
Reception meetings		
Audit meetings		
Critical incident meetings		
Clinical meetings		
Computer meetings		
Management meetings		
Others		

Do your meetings involve one- or two-way communication? At one-to-one meetings such as an appraisal, the employee does most of the talking; the manager supports, questions, summarises and reviews. However, during team meetings, the workers review their performance together and iron out any problems. Communication is two way, with the manager directing and informing, and the employees advising, suggesting and problem solving. Chairing skills are important here – the communication channels have to be controlled so that the most talkative staff member does not claim all the space. Everyone needs to be encouraged to contribute. Listening skills are important too – here is a space for people to air their views. Larger meetings may be unidirectional, as information is passed one way only.

Meetings management

Well-planned and assertively managed meetings are an organisation's most valuable means of communication – they considerably ease the task of coordinating the activities of large and diverse organisations like the health service. Some common themes in unproductive meetings[12] are attributed to ineffective, unassertive control – of people and of time. *See* Chapter 6, Teams, groups and facilitation, in Section 2 for more information on recognising group characters and how their behaviours can disrupt meetings. All negative behaviours need to be challenged assertively for the sake of the whole team. Diffuse the negative aspects of the following behaviours.

---

12 Martin V. Meetings management. *Practice Manager.* 2001 Dec/Jan.

➤ **If the chair is ignored.** The chair has to demonstrate control of the meeting. A fine balance has to be achieved: if you are too passive you are seen to have lost control, but if you are too domineering you are seen to have wrested control but sacrificed the democratic process.

➤ **If a member comes up with an obviously incorrect comment.** Your intention is not to humiliate, so try, 'That's one way of looking at it', and then add 'Can we reconcile that with the situation we're discussing here?'.

➤ **If you are asked for your opinion.** Are you being put you on the spot or asked to support a particular view?
  – Never take sides.
  – Avoid solving people's problems for them.
  – Confirm that your view is relatively unimportant compared with that of the rest of the group.
  – Try to determine the reason your opinion was sought: 'Let's get some views from the rest of the group.'

➤ **If someone is openly argumentative.** They could be a habitual heckler, or they may normally be good-natured but are upset by current events.
  – Keep your own temper firmly in check.
  – Calm the group.
  – Try to find merit in one of the points.
  – Move on to something else.
  – Turn to the group and let them correct or reject the statement.

➤ **If they are over-talkative.** They could be exceptionally well-informed and anxious to receive recognition for this, or simply be naturally garrulous.
  – Never be hostile or sarcastic.
  – Slow them down with some difficult questions.
  – Interrupt with: 'That's an interesting point. Let's see what the rest of the group thinks.'

➤ **If they are inarticulate.** They may lack the ability to put thoughts into comprehensible words.
  – Do not say: 'What you mean is …' It is better to say: 'Let me summarise that.'
  – Restate the point in clearer language without altering the content.

➤ **If they will not talk.** Your reaction will depend on the motivation: are they bored, do they feel superior, or are they too timid to contribute?
  – Arouse their interest by asking their opinion.
  – If they are the superior type, ask for their view after indicating the respect held for their experience. Take care not to overdo this, as the rest of the group may resent it.
  – If they are sensitive and nervous, compliment them sincerely the first time they make a contribution.

➤ **The rambler** talks about everything except the subject under discussion, and may use far-fetched analogies or lose the thread of what is happening. When such people stop for breath:
  – thank them and refocus their attention by summarising the relevant points
  – glance obtrusively at your watch.
➤ **There is a personality clash.** This can factionalise your group and severely hamper discussion.
  – Emphasise points of agreement.
  – Draw attention back to the point of the meeting.
  – Cut across the argument with direct questions on the topic.
  – Restate group boundaries: 'We need to keep personalities and judgements out of the discussion.'
➤ **The obstinate group member** has not seen your point or perhaps is prejudiced and will not budge.
  – Throw the view to the group and encourage him or her to comment briefly on it.
  – Tell the person that time is short and that, while you will be glad to discuss it later, you would like him or her to accept the group's view for the moment.
➤ **The griper** may have a legitimate complaint that is strongly felt, although it may be a pet peeve.
  – Reiterate the objective of the discussion and the time pressures on the meeting.
  – Point out the constraints under which everyone is operating.
  – Suggest that he or she discusses the problem with you privately or raise the issue in a more appropriate forum.
➤ **Someone who has missed the point.** Take the blame and say: 'Something I said must have led you off the subject. This is what we should be discussing …'
➤ **Side conversation.**
  – Do not order those involved to be quiet.
  – Call them by name, restate the last opinion expressed by the group and ask their opinion of it.

A *good manager* will *hold a boundary*, *keep to time* and *tightly manage* meetings.
➤ Meetings often contract (or expand) to fill the time allotted. Shorten them.
➤ Give incentives to stay on target: meet before lunch or during late afternoon.
➤ Review the frequency and duration of meetings.
➤ Use definite times/meetings for discussing routine matters with others.
➤ Start and finish on time, and never relay the meeting for latecomers.

➤ Postpone or delegate topics that need further discussion or research.
➤ Produce action minutes with name and deadline.
➤ Only speak if you have a real contribution to make.
➤ Avoid all meetings that do not run smoothly.
➤ Delegate housekeeping responsibilities.
➤ Use a skilled, firm and authoritative chair. Interrupt people who:
    – begin philosophical discussions
    – tell long-winded jokes or anecdotes
    – rehearse or replay meetings without reference to the agenda or
      minutes.
➤ Ask 'Why are we meeting?'. If an agenda cannot be produced, there is no
  meeting.

If you are *presenting a paper* at a meeting:
➤ keep it brief, preferably one side of A4
➤ use bullet points to summarise text
➤ use coloured graphics or tables to illustrate concepts or massed
  information
➤ circulate copies for everyone to read before the meeting
➤ highlight individual responsibilities or action points for each participant.

EXERCISE 1

How effectively do you manage your meetings?

For each factor, circle the number that most represents your view of your own
management of the meetings that you chair.

1	I spend the minimum amount of time in meetings and they are effective and well planned.	1 2 3 4 5	I spend far too much time in meetings and mainly they could be more effective.
2	I always plan ahead and clearly define the purpose of my meeting.	1 2 3 4 5	I rarely plan my meetings in advance and the purpose is probably unclear.
3	I always establish in my own mind that my meetings are cost-effective.	1 2 3 4 5	I very rarely attempt to establish whether my meetings are cost-effective.
4	I always try to keep my meetings to the minimum number of relevant people.	1 2 3 4 5	Probably my meetings have too many people and not all those people are necessarily relevant.

5	I always publish an agenda in advance and I spend time thinking carefully about my agenda.	1 2 3 4 5	I rarely publish an agenda and probably my agendas are weak and sketchy.
6	Normally people are well prepared for my meetings.	1 2 3 4 5	I always have the common complaint that people are not well prepared for my meetings.
7	I always publish the *finish* time and allocate time properly to each agenda item.	1 2 3 4 5	I rarely publish a *finish* time and probably my time management could be improved fairly substantially.
8	I am very conscious of the need for good a chair and I actively try to improve my skills.	1 2 3 4 5	I am afraid that my chairing is haphazard.
9	At the end of each meeting I allocate time to summarising, and ensure that all actions are accountable.	1 2 3 4 5	I often end a meeting without ensuring that actions are clearly accountable.
10	I always try to ensure that meetings where I am not chair are properly managed.	1 2 3 4 5	Other people's meetings are their responsibility.

If you selected lower numbers, you show good awareness that meetings need assertive management: you are conscious of the need to ensure good performance. Higher numbers need attention – your meetings will be low in effectiveness and not particularly productive for you or the participants. A consistent choice of 5s means that you are wasting your own and everybody else's time in your meetings: almost certainly, the output of your meetings is very erratic.

COMMUNICATION MANAGEMENT

Managers should have in place strategies for clearly communicating the function and responsibilities within each job and managing the risk of staff failing to perform. In all large organisations, policies are in place to observe current and future employment legislation and legal requirements. In smaller organisations such as general practice, these may need developing.

Outward communication skills are becoming significant in all management roles, with managers needing to be public relations and marketing experts too. All employees are ambassadors for their organisation, and outward appearances count. Your part of the organisation may have a mission statement, where the management and staff values are spelt out. This, and any publicised standards displayed in any literature or on a website, will be the image the public expects. It is important to work at these standards otherwise cynicism will set in; it is important the values are adhered too and shown to be working from the top.

Improve communication

Consider using some of the following methods to address any demonstrable communication difficulties. Aim to bring together staff and the public with an objective to seek common understandings and a shared vision of quality. For example, in auditing an operational system such as the phone, evaluate qualitatively, using a soft systems approach such as 'rich pictures' as a starting point.[13] This is a useful approach which helps to provide a framework to deal with the kind of messy, problem situations that lack a formal problem definition.

➤ Draw your present phone system, noting any breakdowns in communications, with a focus on people's roles, conflicts and problems. Is there chaos and miscommunication or order and structure?

➤ Collate information and ideas from others. What are the issues of concern, what visions do they have, are these visions shared? Use the data to support your own observations.

➤ Construct a *quantitative* analysis using a patient/client questionnaire. Ask people how they experience the service, and what they would like to see change.

➤ Begin to think more widely around the issue.
  – What external pressures are shaping the organisation?
  – Who – the public, staff, doctors – holds the power?
  – Where is the conflict and the co-operation between the parties?
  – Who is dependent on whom?
  – Who has the power to sabotage?

The answers to this may help to shape your recommendations. Established and previously understood relationships are changing in the health sector: health service reforms have shifted the power base from doctors and their staff to the patients – who are resisting dependence. Patients are more confident about asking for what they want, both in the type of service received and the shape, or quality, of that service. Teams are having to develop new relationships with their customers.

There are other, more subtle relationships to address: the balances of power between staff and, in general practice, between the staff and their employers,

---

13 Checkland PB, Poulter J. *Learning for Action: a short definitive account of soft systems methodology and its use for practitioners, teachers and students.* John Wiley & Sons; 2006. Checkland PB. *Systems Thinking, Systems Practice.* John Wiley & Sons; 1981 (revised ed. 1999).

the doctors – the influence of more invasive internal and external management present a new and challenging dynamic. There is a new and developing relationship between the managers of healthcare and the clinicians: different roles, shifting attitudes, an emerging power base that is challenging to clinicians.

Look in further detail at your picture and develop a picture of your ideal, compared with the reality. Where is communication breaking down? Where is customer focus lacking? Does your system meet the expected quality standards?[14]

➤ Accessible?

➤ Equitable?

➤ Relevant to need? Is there a discrepancy here between the organisation and the public's definition of need? Do patients expect the general practice to provide an emergency service for what the practice perceives as self-limiting illnesses?

➤ Efficient? Do you deliver within available resources?

➤ Effective? Is the service benefiting both client groups?

Make recommendations

How can your organisation make the changes to meet the standards now required of it? This audit may well identify other quality issues that need to be addressed. Quality does cost, but, as we have seen, the costs of not addressing it in a committed and systematic way are high. Practices that conduct audits in this way are already investing in a total quality management approach through attempting to control and monitor the process and to prevent problems through a systematic audit process (quality assurance). A quality management philosophy requires the commitment and involvement of everyone in the organisation.

Control and regulation in general practice is problematic precisely because of the difficulty of (making and) maintaining agreement, as everyone tends to hold different judgements about acceptability. Hence the need to have an open debate, and then develop agreed standardised procedures.

➤ Put in place some workable solutions to the current problem, for example, who mans the phone at peak times, more direct lines, results only line?

➤ Audit other operational systems within the practice that involve patient services (e.g. repeat prescriptions, appointments) and remediate by recommending some robust, cost-effective and workable suggestions.

KEY POINTS

➤ Excellent communication skills are especially important for those in leadership positions as these skills assist them to make discoveries about

---

14 Maxwell R. Quality assessment in health. *BMJ*. 1984; **288**: 1470–2.

themselves and others; solve problems; manage conflict, emotion and anger; question their position; and adapt, change and grow.

➤ The interpersonal communication skills needed for management include motivating, leading, listening, instructing, organising; writing, presenting, chairing, counselling; facilitating, supervising, delegating, interviewing, appraising.

➤ The language element is perhaps not as crucial as we thought. Words and symbols have different meanings among different cultures. Humour may help or hinder; gestures can be misinterpreted. Facial expressions, timing and speed, body language, word choice, tone of voice and proximics all play a part.

➤ An individual's personality, history, motivation and personal development all affect the way he or she hears and receives information transmitted by another – these all affect communication accuracy. Some other less visible factors also have a big influence, such as the organisational structure and the interpersonal power imbalances within.

➤ Barriers to effective communication are use of jargon, poor listening, lack of feedback, limited respect, assumptions, motivation and confidence. Controlling and evaluating behaviour does not help.

➤ Healthy organisations seem to be strongly influenced by humanistic psychology, where openness, trust and belief in individual growth are paramount; where the management style is open, reflective, listening and interested.

Good communicators:
➤ read the situation
➤ engage attention
➤ make the meaning clear
➤ tell the story
➤ look for clues
➤ check understanding
➤ say what is on their mind
➤ summarise.

➤ Listen actively: paraphrase, ask questions, allow feelings; do not advise, judge or interrupt. Avoid discriminating language. Dealing with racist/ sexist or offensive language is about having the courage not to let it go unchallenged.

➤ Best practice shows us organisations where the decision making is devolved down and ideas are fed up.

➤ Some common themes in unproductive meetings are attributed to ineffective, unassertive control – of people and of time. A good manager will hold a boundary, keep to time and listen actively: paraphrase, ask questions, allow feelings.

FURTHER READING

Armson R, Paton R, editors. *Organisations: cases, issues, concepts*. Paul Chapman Publishing Ltd/Open University; 1994.

Department of Health. *The Patient's Charter*. Department of Health; 1991.

Department of Health. *Working for Patients*. Cm. 555. Department of Health; 1989.

Doanabedian A. *The Definition of Quality and Approaches to its Assessment*. Health Administration Press; 1980.

Ovretveit J. *Health Service Quality: an introduction to quality methods for health services*. Blackwell Scientific; 1992.

Peter T, Waterman N. *A Passion for Excellence*. Fontana/Collins; 1985.

CHAPTER 5

Understanding others

'There are always three sides to a story: yours, theirs and the real truth.'[1]

Fatima Whitbread

Good communicators understand and acknowledge personality differences and adapt their communication styles accordingly: they are emotionally intelligent.[2] What is it that makes people respond in particular, and sometimes maladaptive, ways? This chapter explores some of these personality traits, and encourages the reader to think more widely about their own personality and chosen ways of communicating.

Personality differences can be a source of either great strength and creativity or conflict, so we, as members of a huge organisation such as the NHS, need to be able to recognise this and harness the potential and talent available to meet the needs of the organisation. Good, assertive communicators need to be able to understand what creates personality differences and also be aware of the influences on their own attitudes and assumptions.

Organisations have their own personality. General practice is often run as a family business, with, in psychoanalytic terms, the people within behaving rather like a family, with the GPs behaving like the father or mother and the staff finding their own family role. Acute trusts have their own, formal, hierarchical structure, while community trusts have their own, often less authoritarian, personality. Think about the part of the organisation you work for, and work out how each team member presents themselves.

1   Whitbread F. What I've learnt. *The Times Magazine*. 2012 Jul 28. p. 8.
2   Goleman D. *Emotional Intelligence*. Bantam Books; 1996. p. 266

EXERCISE 1

> **Who, within your team, acts out the roles of:**
> ➤ the father
> ➤ the mother
> ➤ the naughty child
> ➤ the good girl/boy
> ➤ the teenager
> ➤ the young adult
> ➤ the critical parent
> ➤ the nurturing parent?

> **How does this dynamic affect the team?**

Or try an idea from systemic family therapy. Use pebbles or toy animals to represent people: draw faces on them, place yourself in the centre and position the others as you feel they are in relation to you. Ask yourself: what is the current position? Who supports whom? Do the same exercise for you and your current family, your family of origin and your position in the workplace. Are there any similarities?

People – your work colleagues, your patients/clients – clearly differ from each other in terms of gender, physique, ability and intellect, values and core beliefs held, culture, class, communication styles, what they want from life, work, themselves and you. It is crucial that we recognise and accept these differences as it is fighting these differences that can create most of the conflict and mis-understanding that occurs in life. People also demonstrate a whole range of talents, not all of which are commonly recognised and developed in the work-place. Among your colleagues you will find a range of musical, interpersonal, self-knowledge, spatial, sporting, scientific, artistic and creative abilities. Good leaders will recognise and develop all of these skills in those they manage; good communicators will be open to understanding the range of what colleagues can offer.

We understand that personality is influenced by early developmental experiences (social, family and cultural), as well as by adult experiences. Freud introduced us to the concept of defences: in childhood, we developed 'defences' that helped us to deal with traumas, and these emerge later in adulthood when we are faced with difficult or stressful situations.[3] If we hold this awareness, we

---

3 Freud S. *New Introductory Lectures on Psychoanalysis*. Penguin; 1973.

will be able to acknowledge that others too will defend themselves when they do not want to be confronted with the difficult feelings again. Understanding the root of difficulties that present helps to take the charge out of a conflicted situation, and helps us to understand ourselves and others more fully.

Some common defence mechanisms
➤ Regression – adopting childish patterns of behaviour.
➤ Fixation – rigid and inflexible behaviour or attitudes.
➤ Rationalisation – 'covering up' of emotions with intellectual talk.
➤ Projection – attributing to others the feelings and motives we feel ourselves.

EXERCISE 2

It is worth considering who in your team demonstrates each personality trait. These can, of course, be perceived as both strengths and weaknesses. Who is:

➤ practical	➤ frank	➤ aggressive
➤ serious	➤ informed	➤ kind
➤ casual	➤ popular	➤ adaptable
➤ logical	➤ principled	➤ liberal
➤ dependable	➤ tolerant	➤ considerate
➤ easy-going	➤ enthusiastic	➤ loyal
➤ eager	➤ imaginative	➤ unstable?
➤ outspoken	➤ critical	
➤ resourceful	➤ stubborn	

TIPS FOR EMERGING MANAGERS: IMPROVING MOTIVATION

A key part of any manager's task is maximising the staff's potential. Most of us could work harder, with more commitment and interest, and produce higher-quality work with the right sort of encouragement. Motivation is simply the right encouragement for us. To perform well at work, people need ability, conductive working conditions and motivation. What is important for us to note is what it is that motivates people. Can we assume we know? Do you know what moves people to come to work, to achieve, to continue to persevere with difficulties? Think about key team members. Again, to understand people we need to understand their motives, what engages them. What do you really know about your staff, and what do you assume?

EXERCISE 3

Who:
- likes their work to be challenging
- likes to be popular with workmates
- always wants to lead the group
- likes to assume personal responsibility
- likes to set and achieve their own targets
- may enjoy controlling other people
- becomes upset if forced to work on his or her own
- works very long hours
- tends to become bored when doing routine jobs
- performs best when working in a team
- carefully analyses and assesses problems?

In order to elicit the co-operation of staff and direct their performance to achieving the objectives of the organisation, we must understand the nature of human behaviour. The difficulty is that the causes of behaviour are extremely complex and poorly understood. Often the cause of behaviour of the person we are observing is unknown to them, although he or she might attempt to rationalise it. What chance then does the manager have? What we do know about motivation is that:
- employee behaviour is the result of forces in the individual and environment
- employees make conscious (and unconscious) decisions about their behaviour
- employees do what they see is rewarded, and avoid negative behaviour.[4]

THEORIES OF MOTIVATION

A person's motivation, job satisfaction and performance at work will be determined by both *extrinsic rewards*, such as salary and fringe benefits, and *intrinsic rewards*, the sense of challenge or achievement, positive recognition from the organisation, etc. People are influenced by several things: the presence of economic rewards, social relationships, personal attitudes and values, the nature of the work, leadership styles, and the satisfaction of the work itself. Clearly, minor rewards are minor motivators but, perhaps surprisingly, Hertzberg[5] noted seniority as the basis for promotion rewards: the length of the employment, not the quality or quantity of performance.

---

4 Fred Pryor Seminars. Practical motivational techniques. In: Fred Pryor Seminars. *How to Supervise People*. Pryor Resources, Inc.; 1997. pp. 17–18.

5 Hertzberg F. *Work and the Nature of Man*. Granada Publishing; 1974.

Hertzberg noted the factors lead to extreme satisfaction:
- achievement
- recognition
- the work itself
- responsibility
- advancement
- growth.

And to dissatisfaction:
- policies and procedures
- relationship with supervisor and colleagues
- working conditions
- salary/status
- job security.

Clearly, managers have to offer incentives appropriate to the individual's psychological contract. In addition, they need to design jobs with variety, interest, complexity, challenge and autonomy to keep their staff engaged.

Maslow's hierarchy of needs

Maslow published his first conceptualisation of his theory of needs over 50 years ago,[6] and it has since become one of the most popular and often-cited theories of human motivation. In spite of a lack of empirical evidence[7] to support his hierarchy, it enjoys popular and wide acceptance. Maslow's basic proposition was that people have basic levels of need that must be met or 'actualised'. He demonstrated that people always want more, and that what they want depends on what they already have. If the lowest levels are met, the next level is sought. These levels are usually shown as a pyramid, with physiological needs at the bottom.

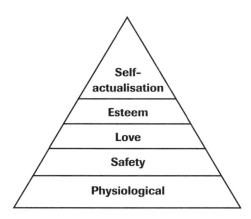

Figure 5.1 Maslow's hierarchy of needs

6 Maslow AH. A theory of human motivation. *Psychological Review.* 1943; **50**(4): 370–96.
7 Soper B, Milford G, Rosenthal G. Belief when evidence does not support theory. *Psychology & Marketing.* 1995; **12**(5): 415–22.

➤ **Self-actualisation needs:** the development of one's full potential, challenge, creativity, achievement at work.

➤ **Esteem needs:** self-respect, achievement, status, recognition in the world.

➤ **Love needs:** social need to belong, affection, good professional associations and teamwork.

➤ **Safety needs:** freedom from threat or pain, the need for predictability and orderliness – or, applied to work, job security, safe working conditions.

➤ **Physiological needs:** hunger, thirst, basic sensory satisfaction – or, applied to work, pay, good working conditions.

This hierarchy is not fixed: for some people, other needs may compete. For one, self-esteem may be more important than love; for the innately creative, the drive for self-actualisation may arise despite other needs not being met. Those who have been deprived of love in early childhood may experience the permanent loss of love needs or desire other forms of nourishment, such as food. Someone who has never suffered chronic hunger may regard food as unimportant. Individual differences mean that people place different values on the same need, and satisfaction is not necessarily the main motivational outcome of behaviour; job satisfaction does not necessarily lead to better work performance.

People need to be asked what motivates them at work. Most of us make judgements about human nature.

EXERCISE 4

What do you assume?
➤ Most people are lazy and dislike work.
➤ For most people, work is as natural as play or rest.
➤ People must be encouraged, or punished, if we are to achieve our organisational objectives.
➤ People like to exercise self-direction and control.
➤ People like to be committed to work.
➤ The average person avoids responsibility and prefers to be directed.
➤ We all like security.
➤ People accept responsibility readily.
➤ People work for money only.
➤ People work to achieve self-esteem and self-actualisation.

McGregor[8] argued that the following was more in line with reality.

---

8 Adapted from: McGregor D. *The Human Side of Enterprise*. Penguin; 1987.

➤ People are by nature motivated and it is only society and the working environment which frustrates their potential.

➤ People would like to contribute at a positive level to the organisation of which they are members, if only they were given the opportunity.

➤ People will only follow leaders who are antagonistic to management when there are genuine, unrequited grievances or a lack of more positive leadership.

➤ Do you understand your staff's motivational needs?

➤ Are these taken into account when recruiting or managing pay and reward systems?

The fact is, people are different. Making assumptions about people creates misunderstandings and communication difficulties. If you understand and respect the differences in your workforce, they will be empowered, and there is more opportunity for you to encourage an increase in personal responsibility and initiative. You are giving individuals permission to be who they are, and this will help the development of better communication between you.

People differ in the manner in which they satisfy needs. The following all affect responses.

➤ Cultural factors: affect the way in which we satisfy many of our leisure preferences.

➤ Perceptual factors: we see the world in terms of our own needs and as our needs change, so does out view of our world.

➤ Abilities/aptitudes/personality.

➤ Frustration: one consequence of being unable to achieve a goal.

➤ Job satisfaction: relates to feelings about, and attitudes, to job.

➤ Absenteeism and turnover are related to job satisfaction, but have little link with productivity.

Make a note of how your organisation meets motivational needs. To improve staff motivation, try some of the following examples of how to improve motivation through improving communication.

➤ Develop a devolved management style: avoid top-heavy and authoritarian leadership.

➤ Encourage increases in personal responsibility and initiative.

➤ Develop more open dealings with staff, and avoid secrecy and manipulation.

➤ Give staff opportunities for brief, frequent, informal gatherings to unwind and relax. Allocate regular coffee and tea breaks. Staff must be given protected time to socialise and relax.

➤ Increase salary benefits: people do not necessarily work better if they are highly paid, but they will work with less enthusiasm and commitment if they feel themselves to be paid below their current market rate. Make sure that people are paid according to their worth and value. Increase the opportunities for change and advancement – people need to feel they have a space to learn new skills or develop other aspects of their creative talent.

➤ Training: in order for people to perform their jobs effectively, to your satisfaction and theirs, they will need training. Take the initiative both to supply and to analyse training needs.

➤ Environment: create physical comfort, and a relaxed 'feel' to the organisation.

➤ Counselling: if you wish to be in touch with your staff, be aware of their problems and what is affecting their work and performance. Offer a counselling role.

➤ Information exchange: keep people informed about what is happening in the organisation, what changes are occurring – new projects, new people. Provide them with the opportunity to let you know their thoughts and ideas about the organisation.

➤ Performance review: people need to be told clearly and understandably how they are performing, their strengths and weaknesses. This stops problems from developing and keeps you in touch. At the same time, it gives them an opportunity to reflect on how your management of them is helping or hindering their performance.

➤ Job descriptions: are the tool by which the manger can ensure that the staff member has a clear and precise knowledge about the job, its responsibilities and its limits – a lack of which is a major source of employee grievance. Define the nature of the job, its objectives and functions. Then set it out in sensible priority order.

➤ Select the correct motivational stimulus in order to reduce the need for continual direction.

➤ The best motivator is the formation of cohesive, well-integrated groups.

➤ Satisfactory hygiene or 'maintenance' factors are the minimum for 'base' performance – wages, security, hours of work, general work environment.

➤ For superior performance, consider group motivation, loyalty, power, companionship, status of person and group.

➤ Note the importance of providing for, and recognising, achievement.

➤ Job enrichment: add vertically to the job to provide greater interest and opportunity for achievement. Allow the worker to plan, set targets and performance standards. Reduce supervision.

Ineffective techniques

➤ Competition: the race for supremacy is counterproductive.

➤ Job rotation: it does not help to move from one boring job to another.
➤ Horizontal loading or job enlargement: more work is not satisfactory – it must be more interesting work.
➤ Reducing supervision does not mean greater responsibility. The employee may feel neglected.

If the organisation does not meet people's motivational needs, they either adapt and seek an alternative goal or they become frustrated and may show any of the following behaviours.[9] How many of these are found in your organisation?

Aggression	Physical or verbal attacks	Abusive language	
Destruction of equipment	Malicious gossip	Picking arguments	
Short-tempered	Sulking	Crying	Powerlessness
Temper tantrums	Fixed behaviour	Isolation	
Inability to accept change	Withdrawal	Resignation	Apathy
Sickness	Absenteeism	Avoidance	Alienation

Managers need to work quite hard at keeping the lines of communication open and keeping alert to behaviours that are creating team difficulties, as they can have a big effect on both morale and productivity.

KEY POINTS

➤ Good, assertive, communicators need to be able to understand what creates personality differences and also to be aware of the influences on their own attitudes and assumptions.
➤ Organisations too have their own personality. It is worth considering the implicit and explicit role played out, and how each dynamic affects the team.
➤ People – your work colleagues, your patients/clients – clearly differ from each other in terms of gender, physique, ability and intellect, values and core beliefs held, culture, class, communication styles, what they want from life, work, themselves, and you. It is crucial that we recognise and accept these differences as it is fighting these differences that can create most of the conflict and misunderstanding that occurs in life.

---

9 Mullins LJ. *Management and Organisational Behaviour*. 5th ed. Financial Times/Pitman; 1999. pp. 409–10.

➤ We understand that personality is influenced by early developmental experiences (social, family and cultural), as well as by adult experiences. Understanding the root of difficulties that present helps to take the charge out of a conflicted situation, and helps us to understand ourselves and others more fully.

➤ To perform well at work, people need ability, conductive working conditions and motivation.

➤ A person's motivation, job satisfaction and performance at work will be determined by both extrinsic and intrinsic rewards: the presence of economic rewards, social relationships, personal attitudes and values, the nature of the work, leadership styles, and satisfaction of the work itself.

➤ Managers offer incentives appropriate to the individual's psychological contract. They design jobs with variety, interest, complexity, challenge and autonomy to keep their staff engaged.

➤ Maslow demonstrated that people always want more, and that what they want depends on what they already have. People have basic physiological needs, and also needs for safety, love and esteem, which must be met before they can reach their full potential.

➤ Those who have been deprived of love in early childhood may experience the permanent loss of love needs or desire other forms of 'nourishment', such as food or alcohol. Someone who has never suffered chronic hunger may regard food as unimportant. Individual differences mean that people place different values on the same need, and satisfaction is not necessarily the main motivational outcome of behaviour.

➤ Most of us make judgements about people we work with, but in fact people are by nature motivated and it is only society and the working environment which frustrates their potential. People would like to contribute at a positive level to the organisation of which they are members, if only they were given the opportunity.

➤ Making assumptions about people creates misunderstandings and communication difficulties. If you understand and respect the differences in your workforce, they will be empowered, and there is more opportunity for you to encourage an increase in personal responsibility and initiative.

FURTHER READING
Herzberg F, Mausner B, Snyderman BB. *The Motivation to Work*. Transaction Publishers; 1993.

CHAPTER 6

Teams, groups and facilitation

Team working is crucial in the caring professions. Most of us work within a team, and even if we are independent practitioners, we are wholly dependent on others to support and enhance our work. In this chapter we look at what groups and teams are, how they form, why team working is important, and how to use this information as an observer or participant to build successful teams and groups, and be a confident and assertive participating member. An enhanced understanding of how teams function should enable us to understand our own role, and work more comfortably within a team. It should also help us challenge conflicts within the team more assertively, with professional maturity.

TEAM WORKING

A team is a group of people working together to achieve common goals. Teams operate across healthcare at all levels: at the top, or macro, level the entire NHS works as a team, subdivided into health authorities, public health, commissioning groups, etc. A trust may be seen to work together as a team, despite consisting of a whole raft of very different clinical groups and departments. At a micro-level, integrated working brings together clinical teams with a common clinical or diagnostic goal, so paediatricians work alongside Child and Adolescent Mental Health Services (CAMHS) and paediatric therapists, health visitors and school nurses, with links to clinical and educational psychologists. And much smaller teams form all the time, to complete specific work tasks, to discuss, to meet and share new ways of working. Team working can help to improve communication and learning, develop a sense of belonging, build co-operation, develop mutual support, motivate staff. Team work generally achieves more than independent working.

There are many advantages of team working. Each person on a team has the chance to contribute their unique knowledge and be recognised for their contributions, and management can ensure that everyone agrees on the objectives and nature of the working relationship.

The way clinicians, managers and interrelated services are working together with specific and shared responsibilities for healthcare provision is still a relatively new approach for the NHS, at least. The government vision of healthcare delivery is centred on teamwork. We have more integrated/seamless care, multidisciplinary team working, and the boundaries between primary, secondary and social care are beginning to disappear. For this way of working to be successful, each professional group has to meet regularly: common core working needs agreement and the group must constantly work to define and agree the boundaries, the ways they wish to work. This method of working is espoused in the total quality management literature. In integrated and effective working, visions are shared and involvement and co-operation is obtained from everyone.

Team working needs emotional and practical investment from everyone in the organisation, especially the leaders. It is easier if the business model/culture is relaxed and accommodating, not fixed and bureaucratic; communication is good; staff are kept informed and their concerns are acted on not ignored; and everyone's views are respected.

Team working is not easy. The team needs to find a balance between the needs of the task, the team and the individual. Do the task objectives fit with organisational objectives? What are the group objectives as a whole? Who will want to contribute, challenge, and who needs authority to carry out delegated tasks? A good working knowledge of how teams work optimally will help you as a team member to work more effectively with the team or group.

Effective teams

Effective teams need each team member to behave assertively, with honesty and integrity. Good teams communicate openly, internally and externally, confront conflict, respect diversity, and problem solve. To do so they have to recognise and value the different roles of members, listen actively to each other, and be willing to give feedback to each other and provide constructive criticism. They also need to be able to appreciate each others' skills. All of this requires advanced interpersonal communication skills, so those teams with assertive members are going to achieve well. In addition, effective teams:

➤ are highly structured, problem focussed and goal orientated
➤ keep clear records
➤ share ownership and common purpose
➤ set clear goals for each contribution from each discipline
➤ encourage participation
➤ support innovation and offer opportunities for learning and development
➤ have external recognition
➤ have diverse skills and personalities
➤ regularly review and process how they are working
➤ agree on common goals
➤ share a commitment to quality
➤ keep the same standards

➤ meet regularly
➤ promote ideas sharing
➤ build trust
➤ are ones in which members are accountable for their own performance, as well as that of other team members
➤ are no more than 25 in number – it is not easy to build meaningful relationships with numbers higher than this.

Teams have their own growth process

Tuckman was one of the first people to recognise that groups and teams evolve, and have incremental stages to their development.[1] Others have built on this work, but Tuckman's four-stage model (forming, storming, norming, performing) has remained in common use.

The progression is:

1 *forming*
2 *storming*
3 *norming*
4 *performing*.

Here are the features of each phase. Those of you who already work in teams will recognise the process.

Stage 1: Forming

At this first stage, the team is tentative. It is newly formed; it explores both the task in hand and the people within the team with a great deal of uncertainty and lack of clarity. There is a high dependence on the leader for guidance and direction, and little agreement on team aims other than those received from the leader. Individual roles and responsibilities are unclear. The leader must be prepared to answer many questions about the team's purpose, objectives and external relationships. Processes are often ignored. Team members test tolerance levels of both the system and leader. The leader's role is to direct or tell.

Stage 2: Storming

Here the team begins to experiment. They try out many ways of operating and relating, with a great deal of conflict, anger and unfocused energy.

Decisions do not come easily within the group. Team members vie for position as they attempt to establish themselves in relation to other team members and the leader, who might receive challenges from team members.

---

1 Tuckman BW, Jenson MA. Stages of small-group development revisited. *Group and Organization Studies*. 1977; **2**(4): 419–427.

Clarity of purpose increases, but plenty of uncertainties persist. Cliques and factions form and there may be power struggles. The team needs to be focused on its goals to avoid becoming distracted by relationships and emotional issues. Compromises may be required to enable progress. The leader's role is to coach or 'sell'.

Stage 3: Norming

Here the team begins to amalgamate and co-operate. It begins to forge strong working relationships, and starts to focus more readily on achieving results, while minimising destructive patterns of behaviour. Agreement and consensus largely forms among the team, and members respond well to facilitation by their leader. Roles and responsibilities are clear and accepted. Big decisions are made by group agreement; smaller decisions may be delegated to individuals or small teams within group. Commitment and unity is strong. The team may engage in fun and social activities. The team discusses and develops its processes and working style. There is general respect for the leader, and some of leadership is shared more by the team. The leader's role is to participate more, to facilitate and enable.

Stage 4: Performing

The maturing team has learned to operate effectively, while still recognising the need to continue to attend to team dynamics. This team is more strategically aware; the members know clearly why the team is doing what it is doing. The team has a shared vision and is able to stand on its own feet with no interference or participation from the leader. There is a focus on over-achieving goals, and the team makes most of the decisions against criteria agreed with the leader. The team has a high degree of autonomy. Disagreements occur, but now they are resolved within the team positively and any necessary changes to processes and structure are made independently by the team. The team is able to work towards achieving the goal, and also to attend to relationship, style and process issues along the way. Team members look after each other. The team requires delegated tasks and projects from the leader. The team does not need to be instructed or assisted. Team members might ask for assistance from the leader with personal and interpersonal development. The leader's role is weakened to delegation and supervision.

Teams can be seen to progress through these various stages of development. They explore, experiment, co-operate and finally perform. This progression is rarely made in a linear or consistent fashion. As teams struggle to cope with rapidly changing internal or external events or variations in team membership, they will progress or regress through the levels. Progress is most assured when teams consciously acknowledge and address the need to develop or tackle the reforming issues raised by change. Teams that do not take this into account will likely regress to earlier stages of development despite the length of time that they have been working together, and this inevitably affects their performance.

Tip for emerging managers – ways to make a team *fail*:

➤ do not give the team a base or leader
➤ keep objectives and decision-making procedures vague
➤ never review the team's performance
➤ ignore the wider organisation
➤ have a high proportion of part-time team members
➤ encourage professionals to recruit, allocate work, etc. to their own profession
➤ insist that each professional group has its own referral procedures
➤ keep each profession meeting separately just as before the team began.

Teams and groups are people who share the same task. Each person working within the team or group will have their own personal and professional loyalties, desires for status and power, emotions, fears and anxieties, and skills, knowledge base, and authority. This combination can be heady, and the group members will do their utmost to find common ground so that they can work together comfortably. As the team forms, it will unconsciously start to develop shared patterns of perceiving, thinking and communicating to counteract these feelings of individual isolation. Group members converge towards 'norms', and anyone who does not conform to those norms will be under pressure by the group to do so. These norms may be overt or covert: they may be task orientated and procedural, such as times/dates of meeting; or, if covert, attitudes, dress codes, appearance, who sits next to whom.

Devolve to involve

A more modern, inclusive way of working is to use teams and groups for all decision making. One or two key people should not make decisions unilaterally. If this method is adopted, a culture develops in which staff feel respected and empowered and the culture shifts from one where people are passive, dependent and resentful of change to one where they are more confident and innovative. Within this, structures and processes become clearer, roles and responsibilities are centrally understood and defined, and there is more control and potential for growth. Results happen and decisions are made collectively, not autocratically or through independent management action. Better communication occurs, everyone begins to understand each others' working patterns and recognises others' stresses, and harmonisation of working practice occurs.

This type of culture is non-hierarchical and adapts well to change. Because the change operates from within, and is not top led, it is cultivated rather than managed; there is an attitude of growth and learning, not instruction or control.

The organisation moves towards a people-centred approach, where people, not tasks, become the focus of management.

Achieving groups

Achieving groups are assertive groups: they co-operate, have a mission, demonstrate leadership and are responsive to their environment. They *co-operate*: through listening, collaborating, working positively, sharing information and feelings. They are more likely to confront issues constructively, having the support of other team members. They work to maintain excellent interpersonal relationships. Such groups are *active*, using systematic but adaptable work practices. They make decisions, consider alternatives, delegate. They ensure that the team achieves its goals, while individuals are clear of their own and other roles and competencies. They use different team roles to contribute to the aims of the team, and balance individual strengths while acknowledging and coping with limitations. The good working group members will regularly review the team experience, while individuals will alter behaviour to enhance both individual and group performance. The group will actively develop a capacity to meet new challenges and demands. An active team will have a shared *mission*: a clear view of their goals and enabled to adopt an action-orientated approach towards their achievement. *Good leadership* enables. It stimulates high performance and is responsive to the task. It supports and rewards team members. The task can reside in one person or be shared and operate flexibly.

Environmental responsiveness allows the team to scan and respond to the environment to identify trends, ideas and opportunities, and actively promote its mission.

In order to achieve the above objectives, groups need to self-monitor their own performance. Ideally, they need to be aware of some of the 'softer' management issues such as group dynamics and time management. Those within the group must continually share what they have learnt. They need too to involve the main stakeholders: the GPs in general practice, the consultants in a trust, the clinicians in community teams – put them right in the middle of the planning team. Use this energy, enthusiasm and lead to give everyone permission to change.

To be successful, groups must have:
➤ autonomy
➤ accountability
➤ authority
➤ responsibility
➤ a budget.

To be successful, they must be allowed to meet regularly, have a self-defined remit, formed and owned through discussion with individual group members, and also be formally defined, with a quorum, agendas and written minutes. Each group should be permitted to set its own objectives and targets, and group participants must be given the freedom to consult outside the group. Outsiders must avoid interfering in decisions and actions made by the group: it is important for the group to own its own ideas and initiatives taking shape. If management are involved, their role would be either as a participant or to keep the emphasis on achievement, positive results, decisions made and problems solved. Through using this approach, meetings become much shorter and more constructive: changes and ideas are presented, actioned and outcome based.

GROUP DYNAMICS

Researchers have shown that groups go through certain processes in their development: Tuckman noted that as well as groups passing through different stages in their development, the stages may not be linear – a group may regress back to an earlier stage under pressure or stress.[2] This is a natural phenomenon of groups, and the wise leader/manager will acknowledge this – not try to prevent it happening, but rather allow the group space to experience the earlier stage and then, when the time is ripe, gradually bring the group back to the present task. In these stages of group development, members may feel as follows.

➤ **Stage 1: Dependency.** At this stage, the group is fully dependent on the group leader to be told what to do. Members will question the leader a lot, and be resentful, confused, uncertain and anxious about their role. Within this, they will be defensive and not take any risks. At this stage, the assertive group member may openly acknowledge and name the dynamic, while patiently waiting for the other stages to emerge.

➤ **Stage 2: Conflict.** The group may begin to feel more confident to set its own agendas, challenge the leader. Members may form internal competition for the leadership position, and an informal leader and subgroups emerge. Criticism of each other may begin, hidden agendas emerge. At this stage, it is likely that the assertive group member will actively vie for a leadership role, keen to support, lead and manage the group through to the next stage.

➤ **Stage 3: Togetherness.** Members begin to feel good about being a member of the group; the group becomes a rewarding experience for the members, with more openness, sharing information relevant to the task. It is a very productive phase, but the group may become stuck in the 'feel good' mode

---

2 Tuckman BW. Development sequences in small groups. *Psychological Bulletin.* 1965; **63**: 384–99.

and not address the task. Communication patterns may become rigid. The assertive group member will be supporting productivity, addressing any inflexibility and encouraging adaptability.

➤ **Stage 4: Interdependence.** This stage is not reached by many groups. Groups perform optimally, with good interpersonal relationships evident, they are task focused and members feel able to criticise each other without it being taken personally. Commitment to the team is high, and goals and the purpose of the team are 'owned' by the members. Flexibility of working practices exist towards individual, subgroups or the whole team. It is a highly creative phase of working together, and one where the assertive team member's role is to maintain her or his involvement in the group without having to address issues.

➤ **Stage 5: Loss/grieving.** Members may feel threatened by the ending of the group or by the prospect that the group will achieve its task and cease to exist. They feel sad and attempt to resist the ending of the group. It is for the assertive team member to acknowledge and name the process, so allowing the group to move on, with regret but looking forward to the next task.

Task	Activity	Features
Forming dependence	Define the nature and boundaries of task.	Group members concerned with why they are there. Interpersonal relationships and boundaries are tested. Dependency on leader develops. Uncertainty and anxiety are felt. Commitment to group is low. Grumbling about task. Behaviour meandering and ineffective. Suspicion of task and each other. Testing and confronting behaviour. Hesitating or avoiding task.
Storming	Questioning the value of exercise.	Conflict occurs. Members resist task and group influences. Arguments about what the purpose of the group is. Members may undermine each other and the leader. Authority is questioned. People jockey for position within the group. Challenging behaviour. Experimenting with hostility, aggression, frustration, rivalry, resentment, opposition. Defensive behaviour.

Task	Activity	Features
Norming	Opening up and inviting.	New roles adopted by group members. Resistance to group overcome. Expression of intimate, personal opinions around the goal are expressed. Feelings of belonging to the group and identification with the group as a unit emerge. Commitment goes up. Defining tasks. Evaluating. Mutually supportive. Showing unity and consensus. Liking each other.
Performing/ interdependence	Effectively pursuing the task.	Group energy directed towards completion of task. Creative problem solving. Roles become flexible and functional. Frequent and mutual contributions. Interpersonal issues now disregarded or sorted or used as a tool used to achieve goals of group. Feel safe and confident. Achieving.
Ending/mourning	Facing the loss of the group experience.	Denial of ending. Termination phase. Group dissolves because task is completed. Group resists disintegration through social contact. Fantasising about the 'good old days' may begin, idealising the past history of the group. This may occur when interpersonal issues prevent the group from accomplishing its task. Bargaining, anger or depression may occur. Group may perform rituals.

GROUP FACILITATION

Good facilitators learn their skill. The team or group facilitator needs to be able to encourage differing viewpoints while supporting the discussion, keeping time and ensuring that everyone present sticks to the subject.

The facilitator's role
➤ Extract feelings and ideas from the audience.
➤ Summarise the content of the meeting.

➤ Help pull the ideas of a group together.

➤ Enable the group to move forward.

➤ Help the group to achieve a successful outcome.

A good facilitator will welcome a group, co-ordinate its activities and keep charge of events. They will follow and accompany the group rather than lead them, intervening only where necessary. A good facilitator is an assertive facilitator.

Belbin, who is well known for his work on personality types, has noted that different personality types are found within groups, with each needing skilful management.[3] Attention to his theory is included here to help the reader to develop their understanding of, and tolerance for, people, difference and themselves.

Personality type	Plus points	Potential difficulties
Completer-finisher	Likes detail. Will complete a task. Can concentrate. Good judgement skills. Meets deadlines. High standards. Very accurate.	Can be pedantic. Poor tolerance of 'casual' or flippant behaviour. Can be over-anxious or introvert.
Implementer	Practical. Systematic. Disciplined. Loyal. Reliable. Efficient.	Can be rigid.
Monitor-evaluator	Able to analyse problems, ideas and options. Good judgement skills.	Serious minded and cautious, upsets the casual worker. Slow thinker. Can be critical.
Specialist	High professional standards. Expert in narrow field. In-depth knowledge and experience.	Not broad minded. Lacks interest in other subjects.

---

3 Belbin RM. *Management Teams: why they succeed or fail.* Butterworth-Heinemann; 1991.

Personality type	Plus points	Potential difficulties
Team worker	Mild. Sociable. Supportive and concerned about others. Diplomatic, flexible, adaptable. Sensitive, perceptive to needs of team. Good listener. Popular. Good at raising morale, reducing conflict and promoting co-operation.	Can be indecisive.
Resource investigator	Enthusiastic, extrovert, relaxed, inquisitive. Good communicator and negotiator. Can think on their feet. Develops others' ideas. Investigates contacts and resources.	Needs constant stimulation of others.
Shaper	Single-minded, extrovert, strong drive. Thrives under pressure. Achiever. Good at overcoming obstacles. Prepared to take unpopular decisions.	Competitive, aggressive, challenging. Pushy. Can be frustrated. May lack understanding of others.
Plant	Creative innovator. Good at generating new ideas. Can solve complex problems.	Unorthodox. Impractical. Poor communicator. Sensitive to praise or criticism.

EXERCISE 1

Note how people behave in your group

Discuss these behaviours with the group and ask them to seek out ways of reinforcing positive behaviour and challenging negative behaviour. Be aware who:

➤ takes initiative
➤ takes leadership
➤ offers directions
➤ seeks suggestions
➤ encourages others
➤ makes helpful suggestions
➤ tries to solve problems
➤ calms things down
➤ encourages compromises
➤ acts as spokesperson

➤ chairs
➤ notes down the minutes
➤ is obstructive or negative
➤ checks progress
➤ keeps time
➤ builds on ideas
➤ challenges appropriately
➤ generates ideas
➤ criticises
➤ offers irrelevant ideas.

EXERCISE 2

How do you perform in a group?

Can you:

➤ work well with a wide range of people
➤ draw people out
➤ produce ideas
➤ face temporary unpopularity if it leads to worthwhile gains in the end
➤ retain a steadiness of purpose in spite of the pressures
➤ influence people without pressurising them
➤ foster good working relationships
➤ lead from the front?

Or do you:
➤ loose track and get caught up in the ideas
➤ talk too much
➤ feel reluctant to join in
➤ retire when the going gets tough
➤ get irritated when no progress is made
➤ hesitate to get your points across
➤ demand things of others when not prepared to do them yourself
➤ show impatience with those obstructing progress?

Some people have difficulty containing the confidences told to them in the group. There is a need for boundaries and confidentiality within the group. Where do you see yourself in this list of containers? Which one would people most confide in?

The chipped, leaky jar	A risky choice.
The plastic medicinal model	Holds exactly the right number of contents and has a child-proof cap.
The rose vase	Rather narrow, difficulty getting things in or out.
The wide necked vase	Transparent. Easier to fill and fairly flexible, but no lid available so contents might fall out.
The casserole pot	Plenty of space, firm, good lid for keeping contents secure when required.
The jam jar	Contains other things already.
The locked tin box	Far too rigid. Extremely difficult to get into. Contents not visible.
The pillbox	Very small container, secure, useful for treasures.
Small, soft leather duffle	Flexible, but limp and rather unsafe.

Good facilitators are aware of, and manage, difference. They work to discover individual needs and try to get those needs met, address and balance conflict, give priority to doubts and uncertainties and tolerate criticism. Good facilitation requires good management and negotiation skills – preparation, management and the ability to summarise:
➤ keeping to the agenda
➤ keeping to time
➤ allowing useful debate
➤ involving everyone
➤ encouraging creativity
➤ making decisions
➤ agreeing on actions.

The ideal facilitator has very well-honed interpersonal communication skills. They know their subject inside out, have credibility and presence, but are not arrogant. They have broad shoulders and good self-awareness. They are patient, self-assured and assertive, but not bossy and insensitive, and have common sense but do not enforce their views. They are good managers – good organisers, particular about detail without being rigid, are non-judgemental and neutral. They can listen and hold awareness of context and group dynamics. They are a clear leader without being bossy, resilient and confident, sympathetic and diplomatic. They can motivate, energise and stimulate, are articulate, direct and clear, and can conceptualise and think flexibly. The best facilitators have the ability to stand back and separate process from content; they are socially skilled, fast learners and keep to time. They do not let their temper show.

Managing group difficulties

Here are some common problems for groups.

> ➤ Not enough time   Group badly managed   *Apathetic*
> ➤ People abuse confidentiality   Too many interruptions   A opts out
>   B is unenthusiastic   Group stuck   Names and titles not negotiated
> ➤ C hogs the time   Members not clear about the purpose of meeting
>   D ignores non-verbal cues   E tries to be leader
> ➤ Working in unsuitable room   F brings up red herrings endlessly
> ➤ Subgroups forming   Boundaries not defined
>   G has a hidden agenda   Group meets erratically
> ➤ H endlessly scores points   Inappropriate teasing and harassment
> ➤ I is anti-authority   J does not respect rules of confidentiality

We have already looked at some ways by which we can best manage groups. We know that it helps if the leader is alert to the dynamics and notices all that happens in the group. These dynamics can be very powerful, so facilitators, as well as the group, may experience strong emotions. Everyone within the group will have their own defence mechanisms, which may make people appear rigid and inflexible. These mechanisms are important in keeping people comfortable and within their 'safe zone'. If what you have to say challenges, do not set out to destroy these defences but challenge gently, in different, less confronting ways: 'It sounds as though you have strong feeling about that – I wonder what it was that has led you to feel that way.'

> ➤ Keep your language reflective, open and non-judgemental.
> ➤ Be provocative and challenging, yet gently curious.
> ➤ Be aware of your own prejudices/feelings and behaviour.
> ➤ Stand back – separate the process from the content.
> ➤ Intervene at the group rather than individual level: 'The group seems to full of tension and unspoken anger.'

You do not have to understand everything that occurs in a group immediately – any significant or difficult behaviour will undoubtedly recur. You can manage difficult groups by:
> ➤ splitting them up, or changing the room set-up

➤ setting a task enabling the issues to be addressed
➤ using wide gestures and voice control – or silence
➤ using a flip chart
➤ have a break or early lunch – then change the set-up of the room.

Manage individuals

➤ Ask them to summarise so far.
➤ Invite them to contribute to the whole group by talking about it or using a flip chart.
➤ Ask them to scribe.
➤ Use individual names as a controlling mechanism.
➤ Invite the difficult individual to contribute to the whole group – or get them on your side.
➤ Use the skills of other team members.
➤ At a pinch – take difficult members outside and discuss their behaviour with them.

Anticipate any problems in advance. There may be a need for a group mentoring: who can assist if a group is not functioning well? Check the number of groups within an organisation: there is never enough time for yet more meetings. Identify the essential ones, then dissolve or amalgamate others. Once the number of meetings has been established, value them and their outcomes. Plan meetings in work time so that staff are paid to attend, or fund catering needs. Give groups a clear leader, remembering that someone will emerge anyway if unelected. Keep groups as small as possible. In a group of eight people, there are eight different agendas, increasing the complexity of relationships and ideas hugely.

Teach groups how best to function. Forewarn them about how groups develop and their dynamics, the personality types to be found within groups and how to manage them, non-verbal behaviour, and the tendency for men to dominate the space. Warn them that oppression rules: the 'experts' and higher social class will dominate, so they need to be sensitive to quieter members and give them space. If members are unaware, give the group some 'best practice' ideas around meetings management, for example, be prompt, no side talking, keep to time.

If the group has problems[4]

Your group has a compulsive talker
Agree to divide the time for a short period and take turns in speaking so that everyone has a chance to give an opinion.

---

4 Middleton J. *The Team Guide to Communication*. Radcliffe Medical Press; 2000.

People are reluctant to talk

Divide into smaller groupings or pairs as it is easier to talk to one person rather than several. Share your ideas and then report back to the rest of the group.

You spend most of your time just 'chatting'

Perhaps members do not know where to start or are unprepared: think about and discuss an overall agenda.

The group feels unsettled

People can be made to feel anxious about giving opinions and talking openly if the group becomes overtly critical and judgemental. Create a supportive and open environment where all opinions can be heard without making people feel insecure or unsupported.

Group members are 'freeloading'

Return to your group agreement and renegotiate your group's rationale. However, the benefits of explaining and working are much greater than simply listening, so 'workers' will gain much more than 'freeloaders'. You should not give up if you feel some people are contributing more than others.

In small group discussion, behave respectfully and assertively. Speak in the first person: 'I think …', 'I feel …' (instead of you, we or one). Avoid sarcasm, taking over what someone else is trying to do and judgements: 'That's stupid …', 'You shouldn't do that'. Beware of giving advice that stems from your own experience. Although it may be correct, it is important to remember that there are no right answers, only a number of alternatives.

Good facilitators:[5]

> ➤ understand group dynamics
> ➤ have excellent interpersonal skills
> ➤ have good chairing skills
> ➤ are able to team build
> ➤ can manage conflict
> ➤ have good first-line counselling skills
> ➤ do not 'perform'.

The *communication skills* required to facilitate involve good listening and diagnostic abilities, and the ability to challenge respectfully. The facilitator's role is

---

5 Reid M, Hammersley R. *Communicating Successfully in Groups*. Psychology Press; 2000. p. 49.
  Argyle M, Furnham A, Graham JA. *Social Situations*. Cambridge University Press; 1981. p. 50.

skilfully and tactfully to welcome, co-ordinate, manage and control the group. To listen, watch and discern any difficulties. To move the group on and to summarise at the end. The role of the facilitator is fundamentally to facilitate change by being open, encouraging trust, eliciting information; to reflect back, approve and validate the group member's experiences. It is also to challenge, to allow tension release through acknowledging emotions, to inhibit irrelevant conversation and side-talk, and to hand over and/or take control as needed, as well as to contribute. For this to occur, the facilitator needs a good, robust understanding of group processes and development.

KEY POINTS

➤ The government vision of healthcare delivery is centred on teamwork. We have more integrated/seamless care, multidisciplinary team working, and the boundaries between primary, secondary and social care are beginning to disappear.

➤ For this way of working to be successful, each professional group has to meet regularly, common core working needs agreement and the group must constantly work to define and agree the boundaries. Wider teams fail when professionals fail to cross boundaries, retain their own procedures and meet separately.

➤ Effective teams need each team member to behave assertively, with honesty and integrity. Good teams recognise and value different roles of members, who listen actively to each other, are willing to give feedback to each other and provide constructive criticism.

➤ Teams have their own growth process: forming, storming, norming, performing. Teams can be seen to progress through these various stages of development. They explore, experiment, co-operate and finally perform. This progression is rarely made in a linear or consistent fashion.

➤ It is easy to fail a team by not giving it a leader, keeping objectives and decision-making procedures vague and not reviewing its progress.

➤ If team working is applied, a culture develops so that staff feel respected and empowered, and the culture shifts from one where people are passive and dependent and resentful of change to one where they are more confident and innovative. If change is cultivated rather than managed, there is an attitude of growth and learning, not instruction or control. The organisation moves towards a people-centred approach, where people, not tasks become the focus of management.

➤ In order to achieve their objectives, groups need to have authority, be autonomous, be accountable for their performance, self-monitor their own performance, share their learning and involve the main stakeholders.

➤ In the stages of group development, members may begin by feeling over-dependent on outsiders to tell them what to do. They then go through stages of challenge and conflict, then interdependence, where groups perform optimally, with task focussing and team commitment. At the end stage, members may feel sad and attempt to resist the ending of the group.

➤ Good facilitators learn their skill. The facilitator of a team or group needs to be able to encourage differing viewpoints while supporting the discussion, keep time and accompany the group.

➤ Good facilitators are aware of, and manage, difference. They work to discover individual needs and try to get those needs met, address and balance conflict, give priority to doubts and uncertainties, and tolerate criticism. Good facilitation requires good management and negotiation skills.

➤ The facilitator needs a good, robust understanding of group processes and development, as their role is fundamentally to facilitate change by being open, encouraging trust, eliciting information, reflecting back, approving and validating the group member's experiences. The role is also to challenge, to allow tension release through acknowledging emotions, to inhibit irrelevant conversation and side-talk, and to hand over and/or take control as needed, as well as to contribute.

FURTHER READING

Adair J. *Effective Teambuilding: how to make a winning team.* Revised ed. Pan; 2009.

Adair J, Thomas N. *The Concise Adair on Teambuilding and Motivation.* Thorogood; 2004.

Belbin RM. *Team Roles at Work.* 2nd ed. Butterworth-Heinemann; 2010.

Freud S, Strachey J, Richards A, *et al. New Introductory Lectures on Psychoanalysis.* Pelican; 1973.

Hunt J. *Managing People at Work: a manager's guide to behaviour in organisations.* 3rd ed. McGraw-Hill; 1992.

Miller LM, Howard J. *Managing Quality Through Teams: a workbook for team leaders and members.* Miller Howard Consulting Group; 1992.

CHAPTER 7

Communicating in organisations

We have looked at communication between individuals and groups; now we take a broader look at communication in the context of larger groups, or organisations. If you are to develop clinically, professionally and managerially, you will benefit from having a wider understanding of where your team sits within its organisation, the roles set within the team and how these teams communicate optimally. All clinical teams would benefit from regular reviews of how their team works, and each member's own role within this. A review involves the whole team, looking at those tasks that can be taken on by others in the organisation. Whatever decisions are made, it is imperative that the whole organisation is involved at each level, and for everyone to be clear about those decisions. This type of review is especially pertinent at key times in the organisation's life: a time of clinical change, a skill mix review, when developing a new commissioning model – any time when the team/organisation is put under scrutiny, especially when it is required to make savings.

In order to undertake this kind of review, everyone involved has to be open, honest and clear about the reasons for change; they have to be assertive in their management of the change; and they have to be courageous in their scrutiny and application of any modifications. Change is never easy, and the assertive manager will have to acknowledge and maybe deflect mixed emotions from those he or she leads.

Nothing happens in any organisation without people. But the study of organisations involves more than just the behaviour of people; this needs to be put in context. In order fully to understand your organisation's communication processes, we look here at management processes, the organisational context, processes and interactions, and people, and why they behave as they do. We take a broad look at:

➤ the organisational context
➤ culture and leadership
➤ the organisational structure.

You will now have an idea of some of the management processes in your organisation, and some idea of the motivations and goals sought by those within your organisation. However, people do not work in isolation. What impacts on your organisation, and what influences behaviour within it? There are four key factors:

➤ the individual
➤ the (formal or informal) group they belong to
➤ the organisation
➤ the environment.

The health and social care sector is influenced by many factors: the 'customers', technology, government, the working environment and facilities, the rules and regulations, scientific development, and financial constraints, amongst others. Structure is created by management to create order, to help establish relationships between people, and to direct the efforts of the organisation towards the goals they have established; and behaviour is affected by these systems.

More covert behavioural aspects also influence how we work within organisations: our own and communal attitudes, the communication structures, team processes, personalities, the conflicts, political behaviour and the underlying competencies and skills of the workforce. It is the role of the manager to understand and integrate all these activities, to co-ordinate, encourage and improve systems and people, and to ensure that people's work needs are satisfied.

Most of us are unaware of just how much work culture affects them. The NHS is influenced not just by the pervading external cultural factors (language, values, religion, education, the law, economics, politics, technology, environment, attitudes),[1] but also by its own internal culture. The internal culture in general practice, for example, could be heavily influenced by the history of the development of medicine, where the values may be patriarchal and conservative, or set by others with different views and values: religion, family or ecological. Those working in such a culture would benefit from being aware of these influences, and noting how far their own values coincide with the practice values. Do you fit in, or are your lost?

These values affect the ways people will accept and tolerate leadership. As flexible, short-term working patterns become more common, people are less likely to feel a need to conform to the work values. The social and 'family' function of work is becoming less important. For some, the picture changes depending on whether they are salaried or contracted. One brings more

---

1 Welford R, Prescott K. *European Business: an issue-based approach*. 2nd ed. Pitman Publishing; 1994. p. 197.

freedom, the other more commitment. As working practices become more informal, managers may need to work harder to support their team in working together to achieve common core values.

THE ORGANISATIONAL CONTEXT

Organisations come in all shapes and sizes, but they do have common factors. There are always two broad categories of resources: non-human (physical assets, materials, equipment, facilities) and human (people's abilities, skills and influence). In all organisations, whatever their size, we see the efforts and interactions of people working to achieve objectives through a structure which is directed and controlled by management. Formally, organisations operate with organisational charts, policies and procedures; informally, they operate through personal friendships, grapevines, emotions, power games, informal relationships and leadership.

Traditionally, organisations can be distinguished in terms of two generic groups: private enterprise or public sector. Historically, general practice is unique in that it straddles the two. While the NHS continues to commission GP services, and they run as businesses, there will always an inherent tension between their caretaking role and the need to make money. However, this tension is moving into all NHS arenas as GP commissioning is rolled out, and all services need to look at the best way to bring money in as well as continuing with their main role of caring for patients and clients. The NHS is becoming a business, and because of this, those who want to develop managerially need to develop business acumen and skills.

EXERCISE 1

Think about the key characteristics within your team or organisation.[2]
➤ Size: small or very large?
➤ Formality: informal or highly structured?
➤ Activities: what tasks are performed? By whom?
➤ Complexity: simple or complicated?
➤ People skills: types of people involved – class, education, age, etc.
➤ Location: single or multiple?
➤ Goals: what is the organisation trying to accomplish?

---

2 Mullins LJ. *Management and Organisational Behaviour*. 5th ed. Pitman Publishing; 1999. p. 112.

EXERCISE 2

Think about these key influences on the culture of your organisation (general practice, foundation trust, social enterprise).

➤ History: when and why did this organisation form? What was the background to general practice /social care/ private hospital development? How are GPs seen in relation to their consultant colleagues?

➤ What do you see as the primary function of your organisation? What is the importance of reputation? The range of services provided?

➤ What are the prime goals and objectives? Money? Patient/client care? Excellence?

➤ Size and location: what are the communication difficulties presenting? What about opportunities for development?

➤ Management influences: are you responsive to change as a team? Is the manager? Anyone else in the team?

➤ What are the routines, rituals and stories told within the organisation, and within the organisation as a whole?

➤ What symbols are used by the organisation and what do they communicate? Any logos, titles, language used that represent the organisation to outsiders?

EXERCISE 3

Identify your stakeholders. Stakeholders are people who have an interest and/or are affected by the goals or activities of the organisation.

➤ What do they want from you?
➤ How do they exert their power and influence?
➤ If you do communicate directly with them, how do you do so?

Stakeholders include:
➤ employees
➤ The NHS and Social Care Commissioning Boards
➤ public health
➤ clinical networks
➤ clinical senates
➤ local authorities
➤ clinical commissioning groups
➤ health and well-being boards

➤ local healthwatch
➤ other providers, including foundation trusts, primary care providers, independent, third sector and social care providers
➤ the providers of finance – public and private
➤ consumers – patients/clients and the public
➤ community and environment
➤ government.

Who do you see as your business partners? Are their ideas welcomed or resisted?

Think about who drives the cultural change, and who resists the change. One of the biggest management roles is successfully to manage change, to ensure we move beyond the status quo, either by reducing the impact of some of the driving forces (enabling the resisters to move forwards) or by influencing those resisting so that they come to realise the need for change. One of the biggest learning points in doing this exercise is to see how far we push change, without enabling people to take it on board themselves. You need to ask yourself who drives the change in your organisation. Who has the biggest influence, why do we resist change, and why is change so threatening for some? We need to be aware of these barriers, in ourselves and in those we manage.

If your team works in a person-centred culture,[3] with a powerful and autocratic style of leadership and management attempting to manage, there will be an equally powerful force within the team resisting this type of management. There will be others within the team who make formal or informal bids for leadership at different times, which complicates matters even further. Or your team may operate as a 'galaxy of stars'[4] – as many general practices run, with each GP making a bid for leadership at different times. It is never clear, either, who leads within this type of team, and chaotic management results. There will also always be powerful internal and external forces pushing all teams into change, which is viewed by some in the organisation as positive and by others as negative. If these cultural forces are recognised and understood, they can be worked with and will provide benefit through a reduction in stress and conflict.

Many teams are not managed successfully and sensitively. There are too many time pressures that lead both the managers and the leaders to manage badly, in an autocratic, chaotic or uniformed way, even if their preferred style might be more enabling. There is often too little understanding of management and organisation to enable managers to manage successfully.

---

3 Handy C. *Understanding Organisations*. 4th ed. Penguin; 2005. p. 96. Weber M. *The Theory of Social and Economic Organization*. Reprint ed. The Free Press; 2007.
4 Ibid.

During a team review, the managers will looking at the tasks that can be taken on by others in the organisation. Whatever decisions are made, it is imperative that the whole organisation is involved, at whatever level, and for everyone to be clear about the decisions. It also needs to be acknowledged that there is not necessarily ever a best or right way to do things – this depends on the task and the state of the organisation at the time. Whatever option is chosen, there needs to be awareness and flexibility around managing both the process and the outcome.

CULTURE AND LEADERSHIP

Leadership styles can give us a clue to the type of culture within our organisation. Managers all have their own individual way of leading. In the NHS, the structure is strictly hierarchical, but in general practice, the *culture* is hierarchical, with the staff responsible to the manager, but accountable to the partners who own the business. If the management and partnership styles differ, difficulties can arise. The power base shifts, staff bypass the manager to clarify issues, and management credibility and authority is lost. This weakens the organisation and can set up uncertainties and confusions as management is undermined.

There are several ways to manage; most managers adopt a style that they feel comfortable with and match the expectations of the people they work for. Each style carries its own strengths and weaknesses, and the reader will recognise their own approach. Can you recognise the leadership style in your team? Here are some examples of each style.[5]

Autocratic management

The people who respond best to autocratic management are those who need clear, detailed and achievable directives.
➤ This is safe and paternalistic.
➤ It carries a clear chain of command and authority.
➤ The divisions of work and hierarchy are fully understood by all.
➤ It works well in a crisis, or in a situation where quick results are needed.

The weaknesses are in the apparent efficiency of one-way communication – as we know, without feedback there is often misunderstanding and breakdown in communication. The critical weakness, however, is its effect on people – most people resent authoritarian rule and respond with resentment, resistance or sabotage. The authoritarian ruler does not respect people and this causes low morale.

---

5 Ibid.

Bureaucratic management

People feel secure with the bureaucratic management style of leadership.
➤ There is a consistency of policy and operations.
➤ There is a sense of fairness and impartiality.
➤ People know and understand the rules.

Although directives, policies and rules are essential in any business, there must be some flexibility, otherwise people react as they would to autocratic management. It is important to be flexible in situations where there should be exceptions to rules, to remember that polices represent legislation for the majority. Ambiguous rules can lead to paralysis. Although it is tidier where approaches are uniform, procedures regular and there is accountability for operations, this can lead to unquestioning adherence to specified rules and procedures, which can be limiting, and stifles flexibility, creativity and freedom. Of course, tried and tested rules and procedures help to ensure essential values and ethics, and help to ensure consistency and fairness.

Does you team work in this way? What do you see as the advantages and disadvantages of this approach?

➤ Clear-cut hierarchies and procedures.
➤ High levels of specialisation can be achieved.
➤ Uniformity of decisions and actions.
➤ A clear structure of authority.
➤ Good co-ordination.
➤ Rational, impersonal judgements made.
➤ Life-long career expectations.
➤ Dependence on rules and regulations.

Diplomatic management

With diplomatic management, the manager takes time to explain rather than order – this has advantages in that people work more enthusiastically if given reasons for a task; they feel respected. The manager is rewarded by co-operation.
➤ The manager has no real line of authority.
➤ The manager is dependent on the skills of persuasion in getting the co-operation he or she needs.

Often staff recognise the attempts to persuade rather than order as a sign of weakness, and can lose respect for the manager. If the diplomacy fails, the manager fails to 'sell' the deal: this gives staff the impression of frank manipulation and hypocrisy, and is deeply resented and resisted. The manager has lost out by not having a clear-cut line of authority – any attempt to revert to a frank autocratic order has an obvious and disastrous effect on people.

Participative management

Each style of management has its own pros and cons, but the benefits of participative management outweigh the cons, as a participative style encourages wide communication, the manager benefits from a rich array of good information and ideas and it improves decision making. People support decisions instead of fighting them, and they work hard to make it work, because it becomes their idea. For staff, there are benefits: people are encouraged to contribute and to develop, they develop a sense of personal achievement and value, and work better and more enthusiastically when given a high level of freedom in contribution. The work climate unleashes power, gives people recognition and a deep sense of personal value and esteem.

However, participative management can take time, and it can be inefficient if used inappropriately. Some people are not intelligent or committed enough to take on board the responsibility it releases. Some managers may use this style as a way of devolving or abdicating responsibility and, if not handled well, it can result in a complete loss of managerial control.

Free-rein management

➤ Delegation optimises full use of time and resources.
➤ Many people are motivated to full effort as they are given freedom.

This carries a high degree of risk with very little managerial control – the manager needs to know the competence and integrity of his or her people and their ability to handle this kind of freedom. It is a level of management usually given only to senior managers in an organisation

EXERCISE 4

Is your team lead management style:

➤ **autocratic:** the manager tells not sells
➤ **bureaucratic:** the manager abides by the rules and regulations
➤ **diplomatic:** the manager takes time to explain rather than order
➤ **participative:** staff have a key input into decision making
➤ **free-rein:** over-delegation carries a high degree of risk with little managerial control?

EXERCISE 5

Use the following task to think again how different people are, in their values, approaches and personalities. Appreciate how difficult it is to adopt one leadership style that everyone would value.

> ➤ I value stability in my job.
> ➤ I like my life to be unpredictable.
> ➤ If I could afford it, I would prefer to be self-employed or freelance.
> ➤ Rules and procedures tend to frustrate me.
> ➤ I like working flexibly.
> ➤ I like uniforms.
> ➤ I feel constrained by organisations that are too tidy and predictable.
> ➤ Rules are meant to be broken.

ORGANISATIONAL STRUCTURE

Here we look at the basic framework within which the manager's decision-making behaviour occurs. Organising, as an activity, consists of grouping tasks to achieve objectives, assigning these tasks, and providing authority, delegating and co-ordinating the tasks. Good managers are good organisers and excellent communicators. They work within a framework of formal organisation, which refers to the more official network of communication in an organisation – that is what the chart below shows; and informal organisation, which refers to the social hierarchy within working groups and the network of communications between staff in different sections.

The number of levels in an organisation is dependent on size. Smaller organisations tend to have a wider range of duties assigned to individuals, often overlapping. As it grows, so does the need for functional specialisation, clearer definition of duties and responsibilities. The type of organisation also has an influence – production organisations tend to be flat, and public service organisations, multi-layered. A clearly structured organisation leads to a clear chain of command in an organisation, which is essential for orderly management. It is interesting to consider some of the consequences of bad structure. First, acquaint yourself with what is considered to be the structure in your workplace.

EXERCISE 6

Draw a picture showing your organisational structure. The ideal may look something like this, with staff sitting in a hierarchical structure:

Head of department ☐

**First tier professional/
clinical management** ☐ ☐

Senior clinical staff ☐ ☐ ☐

First line clinical staff ☐ ☐ ☐ ☐

**Basic grade newly
qualified practitioners** ☐ ☐ ☐

Support practitioners ☐ ☐ ☐ ☐

Write in where each staff member belongs. Then draw the reality. In most trusts, where the organisational structure is hierarchical, people's roles and leadership are clearly defined. However, the structure might be very different within a team, and weak management or weak leadership can have a massive impact.

What are the consequences of badly designed structure?

Researchers point out that there are a number of problems that mark the struggling organisation,[6] all of which lead to rising costs as well as an unhappy workforce. Here are some of the communication failures and their impact on the organisation.

➤ Inconsistent and arbitrary decisions.
➤ Poor delegation.
➤ No job descriptions.
➤ No appraisal system or formal assessment of performance.
➤ Poor support systems for managers and supervisors.
➤ Management not visible and accessible.
➤ Management information, especially financial, poorly communicated.
➤ People do not feel free to talk.

---

6 Child J. *Organisation: a guide to problems and practice.* 2nd ed. Paul Chapman Publishing; 1988. p. 56. Culmsee P, Awati K. *The Heretic's Guide to Best Practices: the reality of managing complex problems in organisations.* iUniverse; 2001. Available at: www.iuniverse.com (accessed April 2013).

Low morale

> ➤ Poor communication.
> ➤ Lack of relevant, timely information to the right people.
> ➤ Failure to re-evaluate past decisions.
> ➤ Poor delegation.

Poor decision making

> ➤ Conflicting goals.
> ➤ Cross purposes.
> ➤ Lack of clarity on objectives and priorities.
> ➤ Lack of liaison.
> ➤ No team working.
> ➤ Breakdown between planning and the actual work.

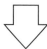

Conflict and lack of co-ordination

> Some other symptoms of poor communication are:
> ➤ failure to achieve objectives
> ➤ low or declining productivity
> ➤ high cost of operations and production
> ➤ low or declining sales
> ➤ high labour turnover
> ➤ complaints
> ➤ delays in implementing agreed changes
> ➤ failure to match competitors
> ➤ lack of awareness in managers.

More obvious symptoms of organisation problems are over- or under-manning, the latter resulting not surprisingly in mistakes; sickness; high stress; delays in making decisions; poor communications; and managerial disputes. The assertive worker is one who acknowledges and highlights problems where they exist, and is not afraid to act quickly to redeem the situation. Our patients/clients and commissioners rely on us to deliver a safe, productive, excellent service. Staff should be free to work in a safe and productive environment, free from stress. There is no room for passivity in these conflicted situations.

KEY POINTS

➤ If you are to develop clinically, professionally and managerially, you will benefit from having a wider understanding of where your team sits within its organisation, the roles set within the team and how these teams communicate optimally.

➤ Each clinical team would benefit from regular reviews of how their team works, and each member's role within this. This type of review is especially pertinent at key times in the organisation's life.

➤ In order to undertake this kind of review, everyone has to be courageous in their scrutiny and application of any modifications. Change is never easy, and the assertive manager will have to acknowledge this, and perhaps deflect mixed emotions from those they lead.

➤ In order fully to understand an organisation's communication processes, we need to look at management processes, the organisational context, culture and leadership structure, processes and interactions, and people and why they behave as they do.

➤ The NHS , for example, is influenced not just by the pervading external cultural factors (language, values, religion, education, the law, economics, politics, technology, environment, attitudes), but also by its own internal culture: our own and communal attitudes, the communication structures, team processes, personalities, the conflicts, political behaviour, and underlying competencies and skills of the workforce.

➤ Formally, organisations operate with organisational charts, policies and procedures; informally, through personal friendships, grapevines, emotions, power games, and informal relationships and leadership.

➤ One of the biggest management roles is to manage change successfully, to ensure we move beyond the status quo by either reducing the impact of some of the driving forces (enabling the resisters to move forwards), or influence those resisting so that they come to realise the need for change.

➤ If cultural forces are recognised and understood, they can be worked with, and all would benefit through a reduction in stress and conflict.

➤ Many teams are not managed successfully and sensitively. There are too many time pressures that cause both the managers and the leaders to manage badly, in an autocratic, chaotic or uniformed way, even if their preferred style might be more enabling.

➤ It needs to be acknowledged that there is not necessarily ever a best or right way to do things – this depends on the task and the state of the organisation at the time. Whatever option is chosen, there needs to be awareness and flexibility around managing both the process and the outcome.

➤ There are several ways to manage. Most managers adopt a style that they feel comfortable with and match the expectations of the people they work for. Each style carries its own strengths and weaknesses, but the benefits of a participative style, if used well, are that the manager benefits from a rich array of good information and ideas, and it improves decision making: a work climate that gives people recognition and a deep sense of personal value and esteem.

➤ Each leadership style is different, and not all work for everyone.

➤ The assertive worker is one who acknowledges and highlights problems where they exist, and is not afraid to act quickly to redeem the situation. Our patients/clients and commissioners rely on us to deliver a safe, productive and excellent service. We too should be free to work in a safe, productive environment, free from stress.

FURTHER READING

Adair J. *Effective Communication: the most important management skill of all*. Revised ed. Pan; 2009.

Bolton A. *People Skills*. Reissue ed. Simon & Schuster; 1986.

Evans DW. *People, Communication and Organisations (management and communication skills)*. 2nd ed. Longman; 2000.

Section 3

Personal management skills

CHAPTER 8

The functions of management

WHAT IS THE ROLE OF A MANAGER?

This section continues the theme of the previous section, being aimed at the clinical or team manager who may be:

➤ new, or inexperienced

➤ developing, or aspiring to, a leadership role within health and social care

➤ working in a small or independent organisation without the support of a human resources department

➤ finding it difficult to work with people and the range of challenges they bring to the work.

This first chapter of the section looks at the qualities required of managers in order to be effective in their role. The field of leadership has evolved significantly over the years. While different theoretical perspectives have come and gone, common themes and principles have emerged that remain important for effective leadership, including the need for honesty and integrity in leadership; the importance of effective communication; the necessity for a solid understanding of the team's business; motivating people; and the requirement to adapt to changing situational factors. Good managers work assertively, co-operatively, confidently and creatively. They work in shared ways with staff; they team build, develop and sustain 'customer' relationships; they use mistakes as learning opportunities; and they encourage innovation in the team. They recognise that they have influence and choice and can influence outcomes. They feel confident giving constructive criticism. This chapter encourages you to compare these qualities with your own, and to work at developing any that you feel you lack.

There are many definitions of a manager and their role but, primarily, managers achieve results through the use of various resources, including people. Management also requires competence in the technical aspects of management, for example, employment legislation, organisational policy and procedures, quality control, etc. Management functions are strategic, tactical and operational. A manager's job can be broken down into four major functions:

> planning
> organising
> motivating
> controlling.

Communication and creativity underpin all four functions. Managers also need to be confident and assertive in their management, to assure results can be achieved.

Planning

All levels of management are involved in planning. To work, these plans must be developed, long term and flexible. At its highest level, the strategic management role concentrates on overall strategies and long-term plans: the organisation plans up to 10 years ahead. Middle management concentrates on tactics, that is, how the overall strategies are to be achieved. This often entails devising and operating short-term plans (from six months to two years ahead). At a lower level, the supervisor's role is to plan work activities, for example, meeting the month's waiting list targets.

Planning needs managers who can see situations as a whole yet can break down the problems into elements. This requires innovation and creativity, but managers also need to be able to be impersonal and analytical when evaluating their ideas: they need to be able to be quick to spot variances. In planning, managers should aim to make the best use of all their resources: technology/ machinery, people, materials and money. Planners also need time for planning.

Organising

Organising can mean either working out the actual jobs needed to be done or giving specific people in the organisation specific jobs in order to achieve the objectives. A good organiser will order resources so that they arrive at the most appropriate time; communicate their requirements clearly, so that people know exactly what is wanted; allocate jobs fairly, balancing skills required against the labour available; ensure that every employee is doing his or her fair share; and know their employees and their capabilities inside out.

Motivating

A topic that has received considerable attention in a wide array of leadership and management discussions is motivation. Bryan Schaffer, writing on leadership and motivation in 2008,[1] demonstrated how the ability of an individual to

---

1 Schaffer B. Leadership and motivation. *Supervision*. 2008; **69**(2): 6–9.

influence, motivate and enable others to contribute towards the effectiveness and success of the groups of which they are members is key in leadership. Without being able to motivate followers, it is unlikely that the leaders of an organisation would be successful.

Schaffer notes four main principles of motivation. People who are motivated are willing to exert high levels of effort toward goals, as the effort satisfies specific individual needs. These people are enthusiastic and energetic: motivation is a personal trait. However, people are motivated by different things: the key for the manager is to find out what motivates the individual. However, while motivation is an important predictor of performance, other factors, such as ability level, can certainly come into play.

Goal setting theory has established that specific, reasonably challenging goals can lead to high levels of motivation. Leaders and followers must work together to establish goals that are specific, clearly identifying the objectives that need to be realised.

The level of difficulty of the goal is also important. Goals that are challenging can increase employees' self-efficacy because such goals represent leaders' expectation levels regarding their abilities. However, goals that are either too easy or too hard will tend to prevent motivation.

Individuals too will be more motivated when certain personal expectations are met. Employees must have strong expectations that the effort that they put into certain tasks will yield task accomplishment. If leaders set goals that are too difficult for followers, the effort/performance expectancy link is broken and motivation is likely to decline.

As managers and supervisors develop strategies for creating motivating environments, they should recognise the employees' beliefs and perceptions. Leaders should strive to gain a deeper understanding of motivation as they work to develop key relationships with employees. The principles outlined above, along with the basic understanding of goal setting (*see* Chapter 15, Goal setting and change management, in Section 4) serve as a foundation for this understanding.

Controlling

Some of the most common misuses of resources in healthcare are overtime, excessive use of consumables (stationary, cleaning materials, etc.), over- or under-maintenance and duplication of effort. In any system, overall, these abuses of resource are the most usually reported. Anecdotally, the most frequently occurring failures to reduce costs in the NHS are:

➤ not using all the workers' talents
➤ not minimising waiting time
➤ not using the correct labour – having highly skilled people doing routine work

➤ not having maintenance rotas for equipment, which would save expensive repairs or replacements
➤ not giving staff precise and clear instructions (which help to minimise unnecessary work or mistakes)
➤ sacrificing quality for quantity
➤ using the cheapest, but not necessarily the best, material for the job.

These mistakes can easily be rectified by, for example, ordering materials in economic order quantities, well in advance of need, encouraging staff to be quality minded, recycling and reusing. Given that staff are the biggest resource in the public sector, managers also need to keep a watch on work carried out for the benefit of a worker or one of his or her friends, and check frequently to note whether their staff are 'on track' or, if they have fallen short, by how much. The manager's control function includes controlling costs and waste. The basis for any control system is to keep systematic records, and communicate this quantifiably and specifically.

The manager has a variety of roles within an organisation. The ones we will concentrate on here are those which require assertiveness and communication skills:

➤ planning
➤ problem solving
➤ decision making
➤ networking
➤ co-ordinating
➤ organising
➤ supervising
➤ commanding
➤ controlling
➤ motivating
➤ measuring
➤ communicating
➤ managing conflict
➤ developing staff
➤ disciplining.

For all this we need to have technical competence and a wide range of social and human skills, as well as good conceptual ability. Here are some of the *recommended communication skills* required of today's manager – mark off those that you feel you have:

➤ assertiveness, confidence
➤ excellent verbal and non-verbal communication skills
➤ good interpersonal skills
➤ leadership skills, able to motivate staff
➤ ability to team manage and understand team management
➤ able to act responsibly, working within the limits of her or his own qualification, within known legal and professional boundaries, being accountable for her or his own actions
➤ able to act with integrity – work honestly and conscientiously, respecting the boundaries of confidentiality

➤ able to act in a caring and efficient way, respecting other's needs and individuality; able to listen well
➤ able to retain her or his own professional and personal boundaries, treating colleagues and fellow professionals respectfully and with awareness and integrity
➤ aware of her or his own ongoing need for professional and personal development
➤ use own initiative
➤ able to discipline and control.

Some of the key tasks required of a manager are:
➤ to understand, support and maintain the organisational ethos
➤ to represent the organisation to all professional and public bodies
➤ to facilitate consensus between staff and their employers, enabling decisions and ensuring that these are acted on
➤ to support the interests of all groups within the organisation
➤ to communicate effectively through writing, reading and presentation
➤ to be responsible for day-to-day decisions
➤ meetings – preparing, chairing and achieving results
➤ consultation – using internal and external resources
➤ negotiation – formal and internal bargaining
➤ developing people – selection, planning succession, training and developing staff, appraisal, counselling, promotion, managing conflict
➤ managing teams – understanding psychology, motivation and organisational culture
➤ managing change
➤ people management – dealing with stress, planning and using time, investing in and supporting staff
➤ taking control – managing the managers, managing problems, decision making
➤ to co-ordinate, implement and monitor within the practice
➤ strategic management – planning and analysing all aspects of the business and recommending options
➤ selling and marketing – consumer and customer relations, prospecting, promoting the organisation or team.

Mark off where you meet the above criteria. Look honestly at the gaps and use this to point you in the right direction for training and development. Have you got the skills needed to develop? Do you want to?

Organisational fit

Self-knowledge is invaluable if you are serious about your career development. Using what you have learned so far, ask yourself the following.

➤ Is the job right for me?
➤ What am I good at?
➤ What type of person am I (a thinker, intuitive, person-centred)?
➤ What do you value in your job? Power? Achievement? The people?
➤ Do you plan for the future?
➤ Does the size and shape of your organisation suit you? What is the corporate image of your organisation? The local image? Globally?
➤ What are the rules within your organisation – will breaking them be viewed as innovative or non-conformist?
➤ Are you achieving the right balance between:
  – managing versus administrating
  – effectiveness versus efficiency
  – overseeing versus doing
  – innovating versus preserving the status quo?

FUNCTIONS OF A HEALTHCARE MANAGER

Which level of work do you see yourself doing in your organisation? Senior (strategic) or operational (supervisory)? Is this appropriate for you, your skills and your pay? How do your employers see your role? This is particularly pertinent for general practice managers to consider. Consider the history: two decades ago, when many GP practices were fundholding, a group of practice managers met to discuss their development and training needs. One of the items under discussion was how their employers saw them – they wondered whether GPs saw them as the managers they felt we were, or whether they were viewed as administrators/supervisors only.

This prompted a survey of GPs in their area. The responses received were varied and, in part, confirmed the managers' hypothesis that doctors in general practice wanted their managers to be administrators, not managers. However, some wanted these 'administrators' to be very highly trained, with the majority wanting A levels and some requesting a post-graduate qualification. Eighty-seven per cent of the respondents identified their manager as a practice manager, 25% as an administrator, 18% as a senior receptionist and 14% as a business/fund manager. These figures did, in part, reflect list size, with smaller, single-handed practices naming senior administrators and fundholding practices naming business/fund managers. However, when taken in conjunction with the qualifications question, the doctors expected rather a lot in terms of qualifications from their senior receptionists. The majority expected their manager to have taken GCSEs (39%), 30% expected A-level standard, 7% degree standard and 19% wanted a post-graduate qualification. Within this, 10% did not expect a GCSE as a minimum qualification, 19% felt A levels were too high and a further 33% did not want a degree-level manager. The conclusion drawn by this group of managers was that, in general, they were managers in name only; the GPs still made all the major decisions, and still refused to hand over total responsibility for management to their managers. Many of their employers/doctors interfered in major decision making in unconstructive ways; very many confused the decision-making process by being indecisive and not allowing their managers the final say.

It is now 2012. How have things changed, if at all? In a survey published in May 2000 in *Practice Manager* magazine, the managers were predominantly white, female (87%), with a mean age of 46.5 years. More than half were educated to A-level standard or above and 53% held further management qualifications. A decade on, a trawl through the job adverts suggests that the majority of practice managers are now graduates, at least receiving graduate level pay, with their employers recognising the need for a more knowledgeable, intelligent manager, who can be much more actively involved in strategic and clinical management. There is an expectation that the manager will have expertise in strategic planning and business development and proven skills in managing people, finances and information technology. Excellent interpersonal skills are required, along with the ability to respond effectively to constant change within the NHS. GPs are looking now for their managers to lead them, to be involved in strategic planning and business development. It is hoped that the GPs give them the authority to do the job they are equipped to do, as sadly, personal experience of working within the medical ascendency model suggests that doctors still struggle with delegation and showing good respect for their managers' skills.

The current role of a healthcare manager

We can see that the role of a healthcare manager, be it one attached to a PCT, trust, practice, clinical commissioning, clinical network, senate or health and well-being group, has changed considerably over the years, and now the NHS is demanding very highly developed management skills. As we have seen, the most frequently occurring problem in healthcare is that doctors often either underestimate or do not understand the level of type of management skill required. Ideally, healthcare managers need to have organisational skills in addition to excellent interpersonal skills, a good level of self-awareness and an ability to research and analyse. Managers at all levels are now much more actively involved in strategic and clinical management. For the profession to develop, managers need to deliver strategically and manage, not supervise/administrate.

Whoever manages in healthcare will have an uneasy task. However well they manage, and however good communications and staff relationships appear, there will always be chaotic pockets.

The manager needs to be able to:

➤ develop leadership
➤ drive radical change
➤ re-shape culture
➤ exploit the organisation
➤ keep a competitive edge
➤ achieve constant renewal
➤ manage the motivators
➤ make teamwork work
➤ achieve total quality management.[2]

Other researchers discuss the elements of management success. All involve clear, honest and assertive communication behaviour. Whitaker[3] identifies *six key points*.

➤ **Clarity:** the manager must provide clarity in all communications, show consistency and maintain effective systems for information sharing.
➤ **Customers:** and staff must enjoy a quality service.
➤ **Confidence:** the manager must be able to increase confidence in staff through delegation and continual constructive feedback, acknowledge difficulties and solve problems confidently, and seek new ways of doing things, taking risks.
➤ **Co-operation:** the manager must agree to work in shared ways with staff, team build, develop and sustain customer relationships, work creatively, use mistakes as learning opportunities, and encourage innovation in the team.
➤ **Commitment:** good managers value staff and recognise different talents. They ensure staff act responsibly and with accountability, and they demonstrate commitment to organisational goals.
➤ **Choices:** good managers recognise that they can influence outcomes, regard issues not as puzzles with one outcome but examine a range of possible outcomes, and transform problems into opportunities.

Good managers expect results. They develop an atmosphere of encouragement, and give praise, guidance, instructions and constructive criticism. They feel comfortable teaching, challenging, stretching their employees. They are accessible and give of themselves and their time; they encourage questioning and discussion. Outstanding managers go one step further: they demonstrate levels of self-confidence that show they believe in themselves and their

---

2 Heller R. *In Search of European Excellence: the 10 key strategies of Europe's top companies.* HarperCollins Business; 1997. p. xvi.
3 Whitaker V. *Managing People (successful manager).* HarperCollins; 1994.

own abilities to select, train and teach their staff. They communicate their expectations and believe that employees can learn to make decisions and take the initiative themselves. They train up the next generation of managers.

In short, effective managers have advanced interpersonal communication and assertiveness skills. They do not just take orders without discussion or challenge, but, in discussion with their own manager, present their own ideas. They are honest with both the good and the bad news, and accept responsibility for their own mistakes or errors of judgement. They praise subordinates when they do well, take corrective action if required, and are prepared to ask for advice and help if unsure. They delegate and develop staff. Effective managers communicate effectively and assertively – in ways that reinforce the self-respect of both parties. The following chapters look in more detail at ways managers and others in the practice can improve their communication and interpersonal skills.

KEY POINTS

➤ Good managers work assertively, co-operatively, confidently and creatively. They work in shared ways with staff, team build, develop and sustain relationships, use mistakes as learning opportunities, and encourage innovation in the team. They recognise that they have influence and choice, and can influence outcomes.

➤ Management also requires competence in the technical aspects of management, for example, employment legislation, organisational policy and procedures, and quality control.

➤ Management functions are strategic, tactical and operational. A manager's job can be broken down into four major functions: planning, organising, motivating and controlling. Communication and creativity underpin all four functions.

➤ All levels of management are involved in planning: strategic and operational/tactical. Planning needs managers who can see situations as a whole yet can break down the problems into elements. This requires innovation and creativity, but a manager also needs to be able to be impersonal and analytical when evaluating their idea.

➤ A good organiser will order resources so that they arrive at the most appropriate time; communicate their requirements clearly, so that people know exactly what is wanted; allocate jobs fairly, balancing skills required against the labour available; ensure that all employees are doing his fair share; and know their employees and their capabilities inside out.

➤ The manager has a variety of roles within an organisation:
  - planning
  - problem solving

- decision making
- networking
- co-ordinating
- organising
- supervising
- commanding
- controlling
- motivating
- measuring
- communicating
- managing conflict
- developing staff
- disciplining.

For all this, they need technical competence, a wide range of social and human skills as well as good conceptual ability.

➤ Ideally, healthcare managers need to have organisational skills in addition to excellent interpersonal skills, a good level of self-awareness, and an ability to research and analyse. Managers at all levels need to deliver strategically and manage, not supervise/administrate.

➤ Management success involves clear, honest and assertive communication behaviour: clarity, confidence, co-operation, commitment, choices. Effective managers do not just take orders without discussion or challenge, but present their own ideas. They are honest with both the good and the bad news, accept responsibility for their own mistakes or errors of judgement, and are prepared to ask for advice and help if unsure.

FURTHER READING

Smith J. *Coaching for Better Performance – what you need to know: definitions, best practices, benefits and practical solutions*. Tebbo; 2011.

CHAPTER 9

Leadership

What do people want of their leaders? One of the ways you can measure the happiness and healthiness of your organisation is to look at some of the key issues in staff satisfaction. Universally, people feel satisfied at work if there is good communication and team work, and a democratic or participative leadership style where staff are consulted and motivational needs are met. People like organisations where the leaders promote innovation, and where training and development needs are met.

Researchers reporting in the *Health Service Journal* have found that staff want a genuine interest in their individuality, a view through their eyes.[1] They want leaders to value their contributions, to develop their strengths and to have positive expectations of their staff.

They felt that the best leaders were:

➤ inspirational communicators, networkers and achievers
➤ empowering
➤ transparent
➤ accessible, approachable and flexible
➤ decisive, determined, ready to take risks
➤ able to draw people together with a shared vision
➤ charismatic
➤ able to challenge the status quo
➤ able to analyse and think creatively
➤ able to manage change sensitively and skilfully.

In this chapter we look in more detail at the qualities required of leaders. Leadership skills, like assertiveness skills, can be learned and developed. Good leadership is crucial as it can transform the performance of the organisation. It is important to look at the qualities our leaders have, and those we aspire to, as leadership style has an enormous affect on those who are led: it can affect morale, productivity and stress levels within the organisation. Teams can only achieve by the co-ordinated efforts of their members, and it is the manager's

---

1 Alimo-Metcalfe B, Alban-Metcalfe R. Leadership. *HSJ*. 2000 Oct 12. pp. 26–8.

task to get work done through other people. Thus the manager, and those aspiring to be managers, must understand the nature of leadership.

All managers have their own, individual way of leading. However, the leader need not necessarily be the manager – in fact, within some parts of the NHS the clinicians lead and the manager enables. For example, in general practice or in trusts, where there are clinical leads: the partners and clinicians lead and the managers *enable* this to happen by co-ordinating the change required. The leader visions, the manager controls. In some practices, some partners look to share the control, moving their organisations towards a more modern, participative and supportive management style; they see the more structured style of management as having too many attendant difficulties. In larger healthcare organisations, such as acute trusts, clinical managers tend to have a bigger power base and prefer to keep the control, which can and does create difficulties for their non-clinical managers, who are disempowered and not enabled to work to their optimum.

The problems with this type of clinical leadership are rife. In general practice, it can be unclear who the leader is: with the staff *responsible* to the manager, but *accountable* to the partners, their employers. Poor leadership structures and unclear lines of accountability weaken the structure, so uncertainty and confusion is set in as management is undermined. If, inevitably, an older partner heads up the practice, he or she will tend to lead with a predominantly autocratic, task-orientated style; and once people assume power, they are unconsciously given it.

In both general practice and trusts, where clinical leads are appointed to head up their section, any supporting managers will be seen as just that – supports – with the power base staying with the clinicians, who may be excellent clinicians but who are unlikely to have any management qualifications. Managers are then often appointed to a position of leadership, but accept an *image* of personal control without the authority to control. They function to personify the organisation, but too often serve as a scapegoat when things go wrong; they may have little influence over either the activities within the organisation or the outcomes, and sometimes additional confusion occurs as other people in the organisation often act as (unpaid and unacknowledged) leaders.

LEADERSHIP SKILLS

New and more robust leadership will be expected as primary care takes the commissioning lead within the NHS. It is hoped that as the NHS matures into the functions expected of it, the clinicians leading the commissioning process will respect the skills of, and rely on, their managers to support the process. In areas within healthcare where there are less complicated arrangements, and most clinical leads have management experience (e.g. within the community), leadership is more straightforward. This chapter addresses the types of skills required to enable robust leadership.

Are you a good leader?

Can you see yourself in the following list? Are you someone who:

➤ solves problems creatively

➤ communicates and listens well

➤ hopes to achieve

➤ has many interests

➤ respects and believes in their subordinates

➤ has self-confidence and enthusiasm

➤ has self-discipline and is emotionally stable?

Office politics and power games are played out in all large and small organisations – people jockey for position, hold grudges, have petty jealousies and rivalries. The most negative of human emotions are displayed – because we are human, and we will all, at some time or another, act out our distresses. The manager will be expected to 'hold' or contain these tensions, and work with and around them in order to minimise their harmful impact. This is a tough job, and one that needs skill and patience.

There are several ways to lead, but most people adopt a style that they feel comfortable with and which matches the expectations of the people they work for. Most move through a matrix of styles depending on the situation facing them. They move fluidly, unconsciously, sometimes finding themselves behaving autocratically when their style is usually democratic; but more often adopting styles consciously, depending on the situation. For example, there is a need to be autocratic at times of rapid and imposed change or crisis – someone has to make decisions fast. A more diplomatic stance can be adopted when there is time to consult and debate.

Each style carries its own strengths and weaknesses, and the reader will recognise their own approach, or that of their manager. Some of the more common approaches[2] have been explored in Section 2, and it is worth recapping here.

An autocratic style can be domineering and over-powerful, and can lead to an equally powerful force from staff resisting management. Challenging the autocratic manager can be hard, as the style can result from unexamined

---

2 Belbin RM. *Team Roles at Work*. Butterworth-Heinemann; 1993. Handy C. *Understanding Organisations*. 4th ed. Penguin; 2005. p. 96. Martindale N. Leadership styles: how to handle the different personas. *Strategic Communication Management*. 2011; **15**(8): 32–5.

defences. Any change can only occur through personal recognition of challenge of this.

Bureaucratic leadership is characterised by hierarchical organisation and delineated lines of authority in a fixed area of activity, with any action taken on the basis of, and recorded in, written rules.[3] Bureaucratic management is safe and understood, but an injection of creativity may be needed to challenge the status quo.

Supportive leadership is related to lower staff turnover and grievance rates, better staff satisfaction, and results in less inter-group conflict; but supportive leaders may be too caring and may need to become more assertive and challenging in their approach so that their staff can learn, change and develop. Leadership that is too directive increases productivity – but only if the task is routine and repetitive. This may work with simple tasks, such as database operation, or administrative tasks, but if this is the only style used, the organisation will not move forward and change. A more structured leadership style is usually the most productive style when managing a crisis.

A diplomatic leader shows an ability to deal with people in a sensitive and effective way, taking time to explain rather than order. This has advantages in that people work more enthusiastically and feel respected. However, the manager can lack authority and is dependent on the skills of persuasion in getting the co-operation she or he needs.

A loose leadership style makes too free a use of delegation: it does make good use of time and resources, and many people are motivated to full effort as they are given freedom, but because there is little managerial control, it carries a high degree of risk.

A style that encourages participation from colleagues is the most current and preferred, as it encourages wide communication and good information sharing, and improves decision making. However, this style can be time-consuming to implement, and thus inefficient. Some managers may use this style as a way of devolving or abdicating responsibility.

Where leadership is top-driven, command and control are the key words: the power base is determined by the owner or managers.[4] Now that the healthcare brief is widening into a total commissioning model, it is becoming more common find people working in a situation where the power base is held by expert teams, not individuals: people who work collectively on clearly defined subject areas. This is a more modern and popular way of working.

Of course, working within a clearly defined autocratic, hierarchical and bureaucratic organisation has its benefits. Staff know where they sit, their

3   Allan KD. *Explorations in Classical Sociological Theory: seeing the social world.* Pine Forge Press; 2005. pp. 172–6.
4   Mintzberg H. *The Nature of Managerial Work.* Prentice Hall; 1997.

responsibilities are clearly defined and change is easy to impose. However, it is not a modern or popular way of working: it rarely uses all the skills within the organisation and is not good for staff morale. Younger staff in particular now demand and expect to work more flexibly, and to have their ideas, wishes and responses listened to and acted on more tolerably. Hierarchical working also breeds discriminatory practice as it only incorporates a one-sided idea (the boss's) of correctness, standards and principles. In successful organisations, devolved responsibilities mean that the power base is held by expert teams, not individuals: staff work collectively to problem solve defined subject areas. This way of working should be encouraged as it paves the way for flexible, innovative working.

Look critically at your leadership style.
➤ Is your leadership style relaxed and accommodating?
➤ Are you proactive?
➤ Is leadership top-driven?
➤ Is the power base determined by the owner/managers?
➤ Do people work collectively?
➤ Do staff understand their responsibilities?
➤ Is change easy to impose?
➤ Do staff work flexibly?
➤ Do people have their ideas, wishes and responses listened to and acted on?
➤ Do you promote innovation and creativity?

Team working takes time. People strapped for time make decisions alone. There is no time to consult. This directive and controlling model results in policies being adhered to, but in some areas compliance is not good and staff are unhappy. The approach clearly determines the way staff may be expected to fit in with the organisational objectives. It is designed to make unilateral management action more palatable. Senior management decide the overall strategy and plan – and nobody else is involved.

Simplistic models of people management seek to direct and control, and see people as dispensable. Best practice shows us organisations where the decision making is devolved down and ideas are fed upwards. The use of 'quality groups' demonstrates good employee involvement, as recommended in the 'excellence' literature.[5] Here, a series of workplace groups are set up to initiate and develop workplace initiatives. Responsibility for creativity and ideas is devolved down,

---

5 Waterman RH, Peters T. *In Search of Excellence: lessons from America's best run companies.* 2nd ed. Profile Books; 2004.

so everyone in the organisation has responsibility for being part of the decision-making process. Change, initiative and learning through trial and error are then not feared, but viewed positively. People are encouraged by being involved and directing the agenda for change.

Healthcare managers need to lead their organisation towards the leading edge of change, by shifting from a simple, perhaps bureaucratic structure to a more complex, mature organisational approach to human resource management.

Does your organisation:
➤ devolve decision making
➤ feed up ideas
➤ use 'quality groups'
➤ encourage creativity, initiative, learning
➤ encourage employee involvement
➤ encourage the habits of self discipline and initiative?

Clearly, it is advantageous for managers to empower their staff to enable them to feel comfortable and confident enough to make crucial and responsible decisions by themselves, without constant recourse to someone more senior.

Changing leadership styles

If teams need to change their present style of leadership, the benefits to the organisation are threefold:
➤ financial: the organisation grows into the role expected of it
➤ organisational: less conflict for those working within the organisation
➤ personal: less stress.

However, change is painful and difficult, and needs to be managed well for everyone to be comfortable with the process. Leaders need to be especially aware of the process of change, and to offer support through the attendant mourning process. When change is imposed, people go through a period of denial and resistance to change, followed by commitment to the change and a degree of exploration towards the future. Managers need to be aware of the beliefs that inform individual resistance to change, so that they can work with, rather than against, the resistance.

Some larger organisations are now too big for their managers to manage everything successfully and sensitively – there are too many time pressures that lead to an autocratic style of management, even if the preferred style, at less stressful times, might be more enabling. If this is the case, it may be best for them to take time out to review the management role, by involving the whole team, looking at those tasks that can be taken on by other leaders in the organisation. Whatever decisions are made, it is imperative that the whole organisation is involved, at whatever level, and for everyone to be clear about those decisions.

Leadership versus management

Fundamentally, leadership is about being able to influence the behaviour of others. A leader is someone who achieves results through people. Leaders are not born: we all have the potential to lead, but no gift of leadership. Every leader has to make his or her own way. All managers are leaders but, paradoxically, not all leaders are managers.

Leader behaviour is influenced by personality, the task in hand (structured or unstructured?), the organisational culture and the team that is being handled. A good leader understands his or her own style and can both diagnose the degree of control needed in each situation and change to suit. Leadership is easier if the team members have similar personality attributes in training, experience, age, sex or other personal characteristics – this is less threatening to the leader. Is helps if you like your team!

What kind of leadership behaviour do you see in yourself?
Are you:
➤ task orientated: directive, concerned with guiding, directing, standards and performance
➤ achievement and goal orientated: wanting people to strive to perform
➤ person orientated: participative, wanting to empower your team
➤ supportive, wanting to compensate for what you see as difficult conditions?

Many years of solid research in health, education and industry have demonstrated clearly that the choice of leadership style should depend on the situation: the job to be done, how important it is to attend to the people doing the job (e.g. by maintaining morale) and the motivation of your employees: their education, experience and willingness to work alone.

Different styles of leadership are appropriate for different stages of a business.[6]

---

6   Clark C, Pratt S. Leadership's four-part progress. *Management Today*. 1985 Mar. pp. 84–6.

Where is your business?	Skills needed
A new venture	Team driving.
	To provide wide range of management skill.
	To have innovation and energy.
Entering growth stage	Manager to develop strong, supportive team.
	Driving leadership qualities.
Mature: meeting boundaries erected by competitors	To ensure efficiency and economy.
	Planning skills.
	Cost control.
	Sound personnel policies.
Very mature: premature decline	To extract maximum benefit.
	Tough and innovative.
	Cut costs.
	Improve productivity.
	Reduce staffing levels.

The realities that shape our choice of role depend on what the organisation expects of us and what is defined as a suitable style: in general practice, a laid-back, democratic leadership style is often less threatening to the doctors; in larger health organisations, a sharper approach is preferred.

Look at the advantages and disadvantages of the following leadership styles.

The prescriber

This leader:
➤ plans, informs, tells, rules
➤ prescribes and directs
➤ makes decisions alone
➤ uses one-way communication
➤ frequently checks on the progress
➤ minimises personal interactions
➤ expects compliance.

In times of crisis, the talented solo leader is effective in overcoming barriers and implementing decisions. However, when these leaders fail, they are discarded. The style encourages staff not to take responsibility for their actions – the problems are passed up to someone more senior to solve. It is not an empowering leadership style.

> **Questions to ask yourself if you are a prescriber**
> Do I have enough information to make a good decision?
> If I were to make the decision by myself, would it be accepted?
> Is acceptance by staff critical to effective implementation?

Persuader

Here, the leader:

➤ persuades people to do the job
➤ sets standards, provides support and encouragement
➤ treats people as equals
➤ invites two-way communication
➤ interacts socially.

> **Questions to ask yourself**
> Have you obtained agreement to do the job?
> Have you spent time getting to understand your team's problem?
> Have you tried to help solve them?

Participator

Here, the leader:

➤ is a coach to a group of professionals
➤ encourages people to solve the problems themselves, assisting only when they ask for help
➤ acts as a *consultant*
➤ shares the problem, but ultimately makes the decision.

> **Questions to ask yourself**
> Who would you would use this style with?
> Have you communicated general expectations about methods and results?

Permitter

Here, the leader:

➤ gives very little direction
➤ provides a general definition of the job
➤ allows people to provide their own structure
➤ deliberately restricts her or his role, provides limited help and support
➤ creates a sense of mission

➤ acts as a chair, for the group to reach consensus

➤ accepts and implements the solution, which the group supports.

Managers acting to support a group of clinicians in their clinical decision would use this style. When used with subordinates, it is very empowering, respectful and trusting.

Questions to ask yourself if you are a permitter

Can staff be trusted to base solutions on organisational considerations?

Do they have sufficient additional information to result in a high-quality decision?

LEADERSHIP AND CONTROL

Do you, or does you leader, tell or sell? Participate or delegate? Research suggests that the manner and amount of control that is exercised in an organisation has an effect on employee performance.[7] Any management system that controls must take into account the individual, social and organisational factors that determine people's psychology. Leaders need to be aware of the forces in the manager, in the people they manage, in the situation being managed, and the pressures of time. Control provides either a safe or a constraining boundary: it either restricts or gives freedom of choice, and it implies something about the individual's standing within the organisation. People feel good and powerful when they exercise control, and exercising this control helps individuals to identify with their workplace. People who exercise control may be more willing to conform; they are certainly happier and less stressed. However, it is worth noting that there will always be resistance to control for those people with low self-esteem and less belief in authority.

Leadership is about sharp interpersonal communication skills. It is about achieving results through people, by being sensitive to their wants, recognising their needs, and being inspiring in your ideas and authentic in your actions.

Good leaders recognise the needs of those they lead. People need to be heard, understood, recognised and respected as well as rewarded and motivated in order to achieve. You can be a more effective leader by developing your own communication skills: your sensitivity, awareness and creativity, as well as your organisational skills. Key management skills will be the ability to delegate, coach, mentor, counsel and train – skills that we will look at in more detail in the next section. You will then be more able to develop your team – the more

---

7 Tannenbaum R, Schmidt WH. *How to Choose a Leadership Pattern*. Harvard Business Review Press; 2009.

effective the people you manage are, the better you will be perceived to manage sensitively and professionally.

KEY POINTS

➤ The best leaders are commonly felt to be inspirational networkers and achievers: empowering, transparent, accessible, approachable and flexible, courageous, charismatic, challenging, analytical and creative, and sensitive.

➤ Leaders vision, managers control. If the leader is not the manager, this can create difficulties: it can be unclear who is responsible and who is accountable. Fundamentally, leadership is about being able to influence the behaviour of others. A leader is someone who achieves results through people. All managers are leaders, but not all leaders are managers.

➤ There are several ways to lead, but most people adopt a style that they feel comfortable with and which matches the expectations of the people they work for. Most move through a matrix of styles depending on the situation facing them.

➤ Now that the healthcare brief is widening into a total commissioning model, it is becoming more common find people working in a situation where the power base is held by expert teams, not individuals: people who work collectively on clearly defined subject areas. This is a more modern and popular way of working. Clearly, it is advantageous for the manager to empower his or her staff to enable them to feel comfortable and confident enough to make crucial and responsible decisions by themselves, without constant recourse to someone more senior.

➤ Change is painful and difficult, and needs to be managed well for everyone to be comfortable with the process. When change is imposed, people go through a period of denial and resistance to change, followed by commitment to the change and a degree of exploration towards the future. Managers need to be aware of the beliefs that inform individual resistance to change, so that they can work with, rather than against, the resistance.

➤ Leader behaviour is influenced by personality, the task in hand, the organisational culture and the team being handled. Leadership is easier if the team members have similar personality attributes in training, experience, age, sex or other personal characteristics – this is less threatening to the leader. Is helps if you like your team!

➤ The realities that shape our choice of role depend on what the organisation expects of us and what is defined as a suitable style: in general practice, a laid back, democratic leadership style is often less threatening to the partners; in larger health organisations, a sharper approach is preferred.

➤ The best leadership style is felt to be permitting. Here the leader gives very little direction, thus creating a sense of mission. She or he deliberately restricts her or his role and provides limited help and support, but always accepts and implements the solution, which, of course, the group supports. When used, it is very empowering, respectful, and trusting.

➤ Any management system that controls must take into account the individual, social and organisational factors which determine people's psychology.

➤ Leadership is about sharp interpersonal communication skills. It is about achieving results through people, by being sensitive to their wants and recognising their needs, and being inspiring in your ideas and authentic in your actions.

FURTHER READING

Adair J. *Develop Your Leadership Skills (creating success)*. Kogan; 2010.

Adair J. *Effective Leadership: how to be a successful leader*. Revised ed. Pan; 2009.

Adair J. *The Inspirational Leader: how to motivate, encourage and achieve success*. The John Adair Leadership Library. Revised ed. Kogan; 2009.

McGregor D. *The Human Side of Enterprise*. Annotated ed. McGraw-Hill Professional; 2006.

Mullins LJ. *Management and Organisational Behaviour*. 8th ed. Prentice Hall; 2007.

Owen J. *How to Lead: what you actually need to do to manage, lead and succeed*. 2nd ed. Prentice Hall; 2009.

Radcliffe S. *Leadership: plain and simple*. Financial Times Series. Financial Times/ Prentice Hall; 2009.

Vroom V, Yetton P. *Leadership and Decision Making*. University of Pittsburgh Press; 1976.

CHAPTER 10

Developing interview skills

'Give every man thine ear, but few thy voice.'

Polonius (*Hamlet*)

The people and interpersonal communication skills needed in all types of interview are multifaceted: the skills required of the counsellor, negotiator, manager and organiser. These skills are first line counselling/listening skills: active questioning, being non-judgemental, non-directive, reflective, accepting and summarising; the diagnostic and evaluative skills of a good negotiator, the skills of management and organisation – problem solving and planning. This chapter on interviewing skills looks in more depth at when, where and how these skills can be both acquired and applied. We look at the application of these skills in the following situations:

➤ the selection interview
➤ the counselling interview
➤ the grievance interview
➤ the appraisal interview
➤ supervision
➤ the disciplinary interview
➤ the resignation, exit or termination interview.

The skills can be applied across all situations, both clinical and managerial: any situation when listening well becomes crucial.

DEVELOPING LISTENING SKILLS

As we have learnt from the work in previous chapters, listening well is difficult. Most adults retain only 25% of what they hear when they are not actively listening. This is because good listening is hard, and requires high concentration and energy. Because of this we, among other things, fake attention; we prejudge – we hold prior expectations of what the speaker is about to say; our minds wander, and noise, distractions, time pressure and our own internal thoughts may interfere. Active listening is a physically demanding, conscious process of attending to what the speaker is saying. Active listening skills are needed for all people management tasks, but particularly during one to one interviews.

A recap on developing listening skills

➤ Remember, we can listen and process information faster than we can speak.
➤ Eliminate distractions.
➤ Stop talking, do not interrupt.
➤ Relax, do not rush.
➤ Be alert to non-verbal cues.
➤ Empathise.
➤ Demonstrate understanding: paraphrase/summarise frequently.
➤ Use open-ended questions to clarify and understand.
➤ Use silence. Do not be afraid of tension.
➤ Allow for reflection.

THE SELECTION INTERVIEW

Selection interviewing is one of the most important jobs in any organisation, and it requires time and energy for both the preparation and conduct of the interview. For this, you will need good interpersonal communication, problem-solving, analytical and planning skills. It can help to sharpen decision-making skills by interviewing fewer than five candidates. Note your personal prejudices and put them aside: keep to the person specification. Standardise the interview and have a system for evaluation of results so as to avoid the risks of bias or the 'halo' effect (the person reminds you of your mother/best friend/an irritating colleague). The following discussion will help either the new manager or one who is working without the help of a human resources department to conduct a fair, organised and robust interview.

Prepare

Almost as much time needs to go into preparing for interviews as the interview itself.

➤ Collect together all the information you require and think about the interview plan (headings or areas needing discussion) and the environment.
➤ Use an unbiased assessment method.
➤ Organise the panel, giving each member all the necessary documentation.
➤ Clarify any outstanding issues with the interview panel beforehand so you present a cohesive and united front.
➤ If you are in a position to offer incentives to attractive candidates, discuss financial ceilings before your interviewee presents.

➤ Aim for no more than three panel members if possible: too large a group can be intimidating and unworkable for questioning. If a larger number is essential, make certain that only two or three members hold the overall responsibility for questioning – others can act as observers and feed their questions into the panel beforehand.

Environment

Tailor your environment to the type of interview, but ensure it is relaxed and equal.

Be courteous, provide refreshments for the candidates and if there is a delay, keep those waiting informed. Ensure that there are no interruptions while the interview is in progress: allow the candidate to feel that they are the focus of your attention.

Conduct of interview

The communication skills required here are informative, open and evaluative.
➤ Interviewing is a professional, not a personal encounter.
➤ Show who is in charge: introduce yourself by name and function.
➤ Outline the conduct of the interview: 'We'll start by talking about yourself and your career then give you an opportunity to ask questions.'
➤ Do not allow the candidate to interview you, but respect that they need to find out about you as much as you do them.
➤ Listen well.
➤ Write notes, which are essential as a record.
➤ Work towards helping the interviewee clarify the various options open to him or her.
➤ Be honest if there are any problem areas in the job.
➤ Summarise frequently. This helps to clarify ideas for all involved.
➤ Make a final summary in which you confirm the areas covered during the interview.

Questioning structure

➤ Prepare and agree questioning well in advance of the interviews with all the panel membership.
➤ Aim to get the candidate to do the talking in a controlled way on topics under your direction.
➤ Keep your own questioning short – the candidate is there to shine, not you.
➤ Start the conversation on an easy area where the interviewee can talk freely.
➤ Ask more probing questions once the candidate has settled.

➤ Aim for a non-directive style, diagnostic and reflective rather than interrogative, by using non-threatening questions and encouraging joint problem solving.

➤ Avoid leading questions where the expected answer rather than the true answer is revealed.

➤ Aim for continuity of questioning rather than disjointed hops from topic to topic.

➤ Use open-ended and reflecting back questions once the initial setting has been achieved.

➤ Reserve the first section for a consideration of the interviewee's employment background.

➤ Ask open questions:

'What did you dislike most about your previous job?'

'Of all the managers you have had, which one did you like most/least and why?'

'If we asked your last manager about your work performance, what would they say?'

The second stage could focus more on the job on offer, and how this person could satisfy the job requirements.

➤ Ask questions that relate to the person's past experience:

'How do you think that your experience makes you a suitable candidate?'

'This job has a commitment to working to deadlines. How do you feel about that and what is your experience of this?'

'I see that you were on a working party to develop a clinical database in your last organisation. What was your involvement and did you enjoy it?'

'What do you feel has been you most successful achievement to date?'

'Have you ever had a crisis at work and how did your deal with it?' [*instead of* 'What would you do if …?']

'What do you feel you have done particularly well?'

In completing the interview, the following should be addressed.

➤ Here is the chance for the candidate to sell him- or herself. At the very least, expect some questions about the organisation and future prospects.

➤ Ask if there is anything else the candidate could tell you that may affect your decision.

➤ Ask if he or she would take the job if offered.

➤ Let the candidate know when he or she will be contacted.

➤ Do not be afraid not to appoint if unsure – you will undermine your own position far more by appointing someone ineffective or incompetent.

Follow up

➤ Contact all interviewees as soon as possible after the interview.
➤ Do not send out the rejection letters until your first choice has accepted the job.
➤ Take up references before making an offer of employment.
➤ Contact a previous rather than present employer for a more honest assessment.
➤ Look at the implications behind statements such as 'Claire works well under close supervision': what is not said in a reference is often more telling than what is.
➤ Inform applicants of your decision.
➤ Arrange for the new member of staff to start and prepare your induction programme.

THE COUNSELLING INTERVIEW

The type of skills discussed here can be used either in one to one interviews with patients and clients or by a manager who may need to offer a counselling interview to an employee whose personal problems are interfering with their ability to work at their best. An external referral is without doubt the first choice for individuals displaying entrenched or severe distress. Within large organisations, there is often a facility to refer employees in distress to an in-house or external counsellor supported by an occupational health scheme. In this circumstance, it is preferable to refer externally, as a clear boundary is created, the material remains confidential and it is easier to separate out the 'counsellor' and employer roles. The counselling interview described below can be used for more minor problems such as persistent lateness, behavioural patterns that interfere with good working relationships or an increase in errors. The manager's role in this instance is to clarify the reasons for the work-related difficulties, before deciding on a course of action.

The objective

The objective is to listen to and give advice on problems that may directly or indirectly affect the individual's work. Although person-centred counselling skills[1] are used, the person that is 'counselling' is not employed as a counsellor, but in a counselling role, hence the use of the term 'first line counselling skills', which we have seen are:

---

1   Rogers C. *On Becoming a Person.* New edited ed. Constable; 2004.

➤ empathic and supportive
➤ non-intrusive
➤ listening
➤ open questions
➤ reflective
➤ observational
➤ accepting and non-judgemental
➤ summarising.

The interviewer will direct or guide the interviewee, with the aim not to tell, but to help the interviewee to solve or come to terms with the problems themselves. The skills used are taken from the humanistic school of counselling, taught originally by Carl Rogers. Rogers' core belief was that every human had within them the ability to see and solve their own dilemmas, without direct intervention and analysis from an outsider. The 'counselling' role here in a work context is not to solve but to assist. The interviewer in this instance acts to provide a sense of choice, safety and positive self-regard for the person being interviewed, while providing a focus of evaluation, congruence, an open presence, encouragement and an ongoing commitment to the interviewee.

The interviewee, if given adequate time and space within which to explore their problem, will know when the work begins and ends; but the manager, in supporting the member of staff, provides a safe boundary through agreeing some core conditions of time (length of appointment – when it begins and ends); frequency ('Shall we look at this together over the next few weeks, every Wednesday?') and confidentiality (what can be disclosed to a third person and when – under what circumstances).

Preparation
➤ Keep a record of specialists who could give help.
➤ Ensure privacy.
➤ Give adequate time.
➤ Check limits of own authority and ability.
➤ Look at the individual's file.
➤ Plan approach according to the individual.

Applied skills
➤ Demonstrate understanding not sympathy.
➤ Ask open questions to encourage interviewee to talk freely ('Tell me some more about that', 'What happened then?', 'Why do you think that is?').
➤ Use closed questions when you are looking to get to the core of the problem or to close the interview. These questions require a one-word or

'yes'/'no' response only ('Who do you feel able to ask for support?', 'When can you arrange that?').

➤ Reverse questions and statements to encourage the person to problem solve:

> Interviewee: 'The baby is keeping me awake night after night, and my memory seems to be going.'

> Interviewer: 'You feel exhausted and unable to cope as you used to.'

➤ Listen, observe and reflect back the interviewee's feelings, as you see them, and summarise for them. As an outsider, you are more able to do this. Note understated feelings particularly, and draw these to the interviewees' attention:

> Interviewee: 'I wish that Max could help with the extra work, but he can't help it, he's got his own job to do.'

> Interviewer: 'It sounds like you are disappointed and angry with Max for not helping more.'

Problem solve: how could we solve this? What will your next step be? Summarise with a positive conclusion and agreement as to future action.

Follow up
➤ Arrange for future interviews to check developments.
➤ Carry out any action promised.

THE GRIEVANCE INTERVIEW
The objective of a grievance interview is to enable to person to air a complaint, to discover the causes of dissatisfaction and, where possible, remove them. Again, these skills can be applied if it is a patient/client complaining, as well as an employee.

Preparation
➤ Find out as much about the grievance as possible – facts, attitudes, feelings.
➤ Consult other people for advice.
➤ Check the individual's file for any previous, similar situations.
➤ Confirm your limits of authority.
➤ If appropriate, check organisational policy and be clear about the organisation's grievance procedure.
➤ Allow for time and privacy.
➤ Check whether the individual is bringing a representative.

Skills

➤ Be calm but positive.
➤ Allow the grievant to 'let off steam first'.
➤ Check your mutual understanding of the exact situation and the facts.
➤ Listen carefully.
➤ Probe deeply.
➤ Do not belittle the issue or dismiss it.
➤ Finish with positive action for the future.
➤ Ensure that you both understand what happens next.

Follow up

➤ Investigate facts and possible causes of action.
➤ Write notes.
➤ Follow up interview.
➤ Take any agreed action.

Dealing with the chronic complainer

For some people, nothing works, but a negative attitude prevails. If this is the case, rather than letting the employee have a contagious effect on the work group, be assertive and positively confront them.

➤ Give them recognition for what they are doing well.
➤ Reassure and encourage them if they feel outdated or overwhelmed with new challenges.
➤ Accept their behaviour if it is not interfering with their performance.
➤ The complainer may be a spokesperson for the group. Check to see whether the complaint or ill-feelings are more widely held, and follow up to correct.

THE APPRAISAL INTERVIEW

The personal development meeting, or appraisal, is primarily about the individual, their job and their development. When was the last time anyone asked you if you are happy in your job and gave you the space to tell them? Clearly, people achieve more when they are listened to, given adequate feedback on how they are performing, given clear, attainable goals and involvement in task setting. That said, the majority of managers and supervisors find it hard to appraise staff performance honestly and confidently. Many avoid giving constructive criticism and fewer still self-appraise. One of the ways to measure the happiness and healthiness of your organisation is to look at some of the key issues to staff satisfaction, and the staff's feelings about their own managers. Universally, people feel satisfied at work if there is good, open, honest, two-way communication, and appraisal forms a cornerstone in this approach.

Appraisals are another way of demonstrating that you believe in your staff. An appraisal can be viewed as a formal system for examining and building on your staff's strengths and minimising their weaknesses. It is a space for staff to assess their own needs and areas of difficulty, and a good opportunity to discuss potential. Appraisals can highlight problems and improve communications. The purpose of appraisal is not to undertake a disciplinary interview, but to work collaboratively jointly to review past performance, assess future potential, and find out what motivates and rewards, the appraisee. They must never be used to identify problems or deficiencies in working, or as an opportunity to re-emphasise past problems. They must never be applied on the basis of insufficient, inadequate or irrelevant information, and as modern appraisals use information supplied by the staff, this is less and less likely. Appraisals are only ever useful if those giving them are scrupulously honest, and present information as opinion not fact. They must be seen to be objective, and always conducted with the information, support and commitment of the whole management team.

The assertive manager:
> monitors staff performance regularly
> makes informal judgements on behaviour and work performance on a daily basis
> notes positive as well as negative aspects of performance
> holds an attitude that most people are well aware of their good and bad points, and will strive within a job to improve themselves
> responds appropriately and instantly to unacceptable behaviours
> sets standards for the staff that make clear what is expected in terms of behaviour
> has written examples of what occurs if the staff contract has been breached.

Everyone makes judgements about their staff, and the appraisal interview is an opportunity for both you and your staff to look at their job and their job performance in a more structured way. Ideally, it creates a space for staff to self-assess, to identify their own needs and areas of difficulty. The objective is not to tell the member of staff what is going wrong; the aim is to support and encourage them to discuss their own potential for development and subsequent training needs. The ethos and culture of medicine used to make clinical peer appraisal difficult, but now appraisal systems are in place for all practicing clinicians within the NHS, so familiarity makes clinical staff less defensive about the process.

Appraisers should be non-judgemental and use evidence, not anecdotes. They should use assertive, counselling, problem-solving and facilitation skills to be:

➤ fair, unbiased
➤ constructive and positive
➤ objective
➤ open and clear
➤ supportive yet challenging.

Appraisals are therefore not hierarchically based, but seen as developmental. They are not performance managed, and are focussed on process, not outcomes. The needs of the individual and the organisation they work within do not always coincide, so if conflict exists this should be explored. Those being appraised need to know what is expected of them, and obtain fair, constructive, objective and positive feedback on how they are performing. Appraisals should be conducted within an environment that is open, positive, supportive and developmental.

The appraisee should be given the opportunity to:

➤ engage in the discussion
➤ reflect on their own performance
➤ state needs and expectations
➤ seek clarification
➤ set meaningful – subjective and objective – targets.

All judgements must be evidence based and sourced: made on the basis of sound information.

For clinical and non-clinical staff, the appraisal is an opportunity to appraise interpersonal and communication skills; attitudes to work and clients; and personal effectiveness, such as the patient approach, communication and leadership skills, any contributions to the management process. Appraises can address these challenges by developing their own personal skills to learn how to deal with conflict, give constructive criticism, and give and receive feedback. The organisation can support this by:

➤ behaving in an open way
➤ developing strong and gifted teams
➤ reinforcing the concept of mutual support
➤ learning from its mistakes
➤ believing in the importance of service delivery
➤ training and developing staff
➤ being self-evaluative.

The appraisal process

Step 1: Monitor staff performance

All employers make informal judgements on their employees' behaviour and work performance. It is important to look at, and note, positive as well as negative aspects of employees' work on an ongoing basis. Attitudes to colleagues and the public are transparent to the alert manager who spends time informally observing. Work well done needs to be praised: thanks (verbal or written) are important if staff are expected to continue producing work of a high standard. Poor work or unacceptable behaviour needs challenging immediately, outside of the appraisal interview.

➤ Set your standards for the staff and make clear at regular intervals what is expected of them in terms of behaviour.

➤ Anger directed at a member of the public should never be allowed to occur without some form of immediate staff counselling.

➤ Develop and follow a written code and then you will be clearer when a breach of conduct occurs.

Step 2: Prepare

During the appraisal, do not shy from being honest if honesty, clarity and constructive criticism is required and asked for. This is easier if the member of staff has the space to self-appraise and assess their own strengths and weaknesses – then your own input may become unnecessary. Once they have identified a point to work on, it becomes easier to offer pointers of your own.

Even if you work for a small organisation such as general practice, it is still important to prepare staff ahead formally. Inform them you will be interviewing and when, and develop supporting paperwork such as a personal development plan, where they consider their past performance, areas of achievement and future training needs.

Step 3: Communication skills

During the appraisal, look together at ways of extending and improving work performance. Allow ample, uninterrupted and private time, and stress the two-way nature of the interview. If the employee is closed to the idea of self-assessment, construct hypothetical situations so that they can assess their likely reaction.

➤ 'How do you feel in the presence of angry, impatient people?'

➤ 'How do you react to the habitual attendee who you feel is wasting the doctor's time?'

➤ 'How do you feel when the doctor asks you to pass a message on that you know will be badly received?'

➤ 'Do you find it easy to delegate?'

➤ 'Do you find all the people who work here easy to get on with?'

➤ Encourage staff to take the lead.
➤ Use open, reflective questioning so that the interviewee can expand on what they think.
➤ Ask for some specifics about how the job has gone that year.
➤ Make statements about performance after they have given their views.
➤ Add to rather than submerge their points.
➤ Listen and observe, frequently reflect and summarise.
➤ Where poor performance is under scrutiny, emphasise 'How can we improve?', without noting the problem.
➤ Make a final summary, emphasising conclusions and future action.

Step 4: Follow up
➤ If you are not using organisational paperwork, complete an appraisal form that identifies current problems and targeted areas for action.
➤ Give a copy to the member of staff.
➤ Note areas that you have promised to investigate or change, and do so.
➤ Set a date, and make sure that any action taken is also followed up.

Giving constructive feedback

As managers, one part of our job is to give people positive and negative feedback so that they can learn and develop their work skills. We also need to be able to express grievances to those who manage us. We can show others within the practice how best to do this assertively so that resentments and negative feelings do not fester. All too often, we fail to give reward, or positive 'strokes', to people through embarrassment or awkwardness. People need to be told when they are doing splendidly; once good behaviour is reinforced it is more likely that it will be repeated. If staff are working particularly well, or producing work of a consistently high standard, notice it, give verbal praise and consider other pay or non-pay related benefits. Everyone appreciates it when his or her work is noticed. Organisations that have formal or informal appraisal systems in use tend to have lower staff turnover and a happier working environment.

➤ Be honest. Insincerity always negates the compliment. We often give insincere compliments as a response to being given one ourselves.
➤ Be specific. Avoid using vague statements such as 'You were great/terrific': these do convey a positive message, but leave the other person unsure about what you mean. Try clarity:

'I really admire the way you take so much time when you explain things to new staff, I can see you have a lot of patience.'

'That could have been embarrassing; I thought you diffused the situation very tactfully.'

'I'm very impressed by your ability to sit back and weigh up a situation before acting'

'I admire the way you put the patients at their ease when they first come in.'

Performance appraisal schemes can also include self-assessment tools such as assessing one's level of ability using a competency grid, or getting feedback from a 360-degree questionnaire[2] – a questionnaire that explores your personality and skills as perceived by colleagues at different levels in the organisation, giving feedback from members of an immediate work circle. Most often, 360-degree feedback will include direct feedback from an employee's subordinates, peers and supervisor(s), as well as a self-evaluation. It can also include, in some cases, feedback from external sources, such as patients/clients or other interested stakeholders. It may be contrasted with 'upward feedback', where managers are given feedback only by those directly reporting to them.

Introducing an appraisal system should be a positive, strengthening experience; it should build on the strengths of both the organisation and the individuals working within it. Praise leads to constructive self-analysis, which benefits the employer as well as the employee.

SUPERVISION

If you supervise staff, or have a practitioner or clinical teaching role, all the above skills will be used. In addition, other skills need to be developed in order to support, encourage and develop your employees, colleagues or students, clinically, professionally and personally. Work through the checklist[3] in Exercise 1 to self-evaluate and also ask your colleague or student to evaluate your supervision skills. The student rates your clinical teaching skills on the scale of 1 (poor) to 5 (excellent), and it is through the discussion and evaluation of these core skills that you will gain insight into the areas that you need to develop.

---

2 Bracken DW, Rose DS. When does 360-degree feedback create behaviour change? And how would we know when it does? *Journal of Business and Psychology*. 2011; **26**(2): 183–92. Maylett T. 360-degree feedback revisited: the transition from development to appraisal. *Compensation and Benefits Review*. 2009; **41**(5): 52–9.

3 Shared with the permission of Ann Parker, MCSLT. Senior teaching fellow, University College London.

EXERCISE 1

> Preparing and inducting student at start of placement.
> Getting information about the student's past clinical experience, skills and expectations.
> Agreeing goals for the placement with the student.
> Giving positive feedback.
> Giving immediate feedback.
> Helping the student develop self-evaluation skills.
> Focussing feedback on specific behaviour.
> Collaborating with the student on their plans, evaluations and future client management.
> Leaving the student alone.
> Receiving feedback from student about own clinical techniques.
> Receiving feedback from student about own teaching approaches.
> Encouraging the student to ask questions.
> Being aware of the uses and abuses of questioning the student.
> Using convergent/divergent questions consciously and appropriately.
> Providing emotional support for the student.
> Acknowledging own emotional response to clinical and teaching situations.
> Establishing a relationship that allows the student maximise their function in the placement.

This list highlights the usefulness of using advanced communication skills in any situation where we are supporting and developing colleagues: when we need to develop self-awareness, humility and constructive concern for the student's welfare. Experienced clinical managers are organised and proactive – they prepare in advance for a full induction and find out the information on the student's expectations and experience. They work collaboratively, agreeing shared goals. They are assertive in giving constructive criticism and they are generous in sharing their own knowledge and skills. They are self-aware enough to know when it is appropriate to leave the student alone, allowing them to make their own mistakes. They are open to receiving constructive criticism from others. They encourage and support, and are aware of the uses and abuses of too many, and too intrusive, questions. Finally, they are aware of and acknowledge their own emotional responses, which helps to establish and build the relationship.

This list could also be used by non-clinical managers, to help inform the ways they induct new members of staff, or as part of a 360-degree appraisal process. Either way, the feedback given should be a positive, strengthening experience, enabling the supervisor to move forward in developing his or her communication and supervisory skills.

Supervision policies[4] can be set up to guide, inform or support personal or clinical practice. The aims may be pastoral, to enable the individual to overcome work-based challenges, or recognise what has gone well, or discuss organisational issues, or provide a supportive environment with clear direction and guidance on problem solving. Clinical supervision aims vary, and may be set up with employees, peers or students, but may include:

➤ creating a learning environment which promotes effective clinical practice and identifies ongoing learning needs

➤ reinforcing good practice and providing feedback about individual case management

➤ discussing caseload management, workload allocation and targets

➤ discussing progress with appraisal and personal development plan objectives

➤ monitoring clinical competencies through use of existing frameworks, for example, professional and organisational standards.

There are various formal and informal supervision models available, including buddy/mentor systems (usually adopted for new recruits); peer support (which can be anything from individual peer meetings through to formal supervision groups, with clinical focus groups, professional case reviews and joint sessions being equally valid forums); one to one with a senior practitioner or professional lead; and shadowing. Within this, the process is usually qualified to note the time and length of meetings, the venues, the paperwork required, and the roles and responsibilities of both supervisor and supervisee.

Supervision frameworks[5] should allow the employee to analyse specific strengths and weaknesses in their performance. Feedback should be goal related (towards clearly specified objectives) and timely, reducing feedback as the person progresses towards independence and competence. It should be positive and liberating, so it helps the employee confidently to assess their own performance. It should be personal and individualised, and collegial/collaborative, so that the person to whom you are feeding back 'owns' the information. Finally, before each session ends, work out together a practical way forward, a future activity which will help maintain present strengths.

It is important to develop the capacity to reflect on action – after you have carried out the action. Central to this process is the asking of appropriate questions – in supervision or group meetings – to ensure that the reflection is used, not just rehearsed. If working in a peer supervision or co-counselling type of framework, it is useful to set ground rules to ensure safe practice. These

---

4 Adapted from: Rowe F. *Supervision Guidelines*. Integrated Therapy Service for Children and Young People, Somerset Partnership Primary Care Trust; 2010.

5 Adapted from: Watts NT. *Handbook of Clinical Teaching*. Churchill Livingstone; 1990. p. 207.

may be formed by the group or the leader/facilitator, and should include clarification of the:

➤ roles of group members and leader

➤ venue, times, frequency

➤ confidentiality agreements

➤ procedures in the event of disclosure of unsafe practice

➤ permissions to record reflections

➤ permitted issues/themes for discussion

➤ negotiation of emergency slots/time

➤ 'rules' of communication, for example, respectful, non-judgemental, solution-focussed, open/reflective questioning, how to feedback, mobiles off.

There may be some general ground rules, such as permission to make mistakes, reading ground rules before each session, keeping of reflective diaries, etc. It is important that those attending are encouraged and supported to reflect on their practice, not ruminate/rehearse the same stories: repeating a narrative can be irritating a best; at worst, no learning is demonstrated.

Dealing with boundary violations

We will all have had experience of boundary violations if we work with people. Each time it happens, consideration needs to be given to a resolution that includes some understanding of what went wrong and why, and an understanding from our supervisee that it must not happen again. Common boundary violations occur when, for example:

➤ staff try to make friends with their patients/clients

➤ payments are involved

➤ there is misunderstanding of roles

➤ public confidentiality is inadvertently broken

➤ privacy is disrespected

➤ consent is not obtained.

Each one of us will have our own example. What makes boundary violations problematic is that there are no automatic rights and wrongs, no clear answers. Whichever route you choose, it is likely that you will be left with uncomfortable feelings because there is no resolution that will satisfy all parties: there are rarely clear-cut solutions to these things. However, it is worth considering, with your supervisee, in each situation:

➤ their personal core values and beliefs

➤ how these values sit with the organisation you work for

➤ the manner and content of what is said, and what this might communicate to people who use our services

➤ what the moral and ethical implications are
➤ how the conversation/discourse affirms or undermines client/patient autonomy
➤ what would engage/disengage the patient/clients.[6]

Consider the challenges, too:
➤ confidentiality
➤ responsibilities, boundaries, privacy
➤ respecting loyalties to patients, colleagues, carers
➤ assertive decision making
➤ consent
➤ cultural issues
➤ moral versus clinical duty.

In each case, where boundaries are broken, discussion with a manager or supervisor must occur, just as it does when any untoward incident occurs. Discussion with colleagues, too, opens up useful, differing viewpoints. In the light of these discussions, the manager/supervisor needs to check that any decisions made are effective, efficient and equitable. Within this, too, we need to ensure that we and our staff behave assertively and with integrity.

Assertiveness and adhering to professional responsibilities[7]

Anyone who works in a clinical setting has a responsibility to themselves, their clients and their colleagues to adhere to certain principles, allowing for mutual trust and respect. Behaving assertively, honestly, clearly, ethically and morally can help us to uphold those values. Managers need to ensure that the practitioners/clinicians they manage understand their professional responsibilities.

1 Clinicians have a responsibility to work within their own limitations

Professionally, practitioners need to be responsible and assertive about looking after themselves. They must ensure that they are appropriately supported and accountable. They need to consider the limitations of their training and experience and work within these limits, taking advantage of all available professional support. If their work with people requires the provision of supervision, they must ensure that they make every effort to attend, as there is no professional defence if they do not push for what they need nor attend what is offered.

---

6 Body R, McAllister L. *Ethics in Speech and Language Therapy*. Wiley-Blackwell; 2009.
7 Abridged from: www.bacp.co.uk (accessed April 2013).

➤ Staff must be assertive about saying 'no' when they feel that they have reached the limits of their ability. If they feel unqualified to provide a level of service, or feel unwell or unable to practise safely, for whatever reason, they must be clear about this and withdraw from working, and seek appropriate professional support and services as the need arises. Attending to one's own well-being is essential to sustaining good practice.

➤ To maintain competent practice, staff should regularly review their need for professional and personal support and obtain appropriate services for themselves. This is a personal responsibility, not the employer's. Regularly monitoring and reviewing one's own work is essential to maintaining good practice. It is important to be conscientious in considering feedback from colleagues. Responding constructively to feedback helps to advance practice. Committing to good practice requires staff to keep up to date with the latest knowledge and respond to changing circumstances.

➤ Assertive practice involves clarifying and agreeing the rights and responsibilities of both the practitioner and the client at appropriate points in their working relationship, not fudging issues or passively being led by another's agenda.

➤ Staff must be proactive, and ensure records are accurate, not including irrelevant or personal opinion, respectful of clients and colleagues, and protected from unauthorised disclosure.

➤ Staff must be clear about any legal requirements concerning their work, and consider these conscientiously and be legally accountable for their practice.

2   *There is a responsibility to gain and honour the trust of clients*

Keeping trust requires that we are always open and honest in our dealings with people, and that we remain clear about our working principles. Thus patients/ clients need to know, and be reassured, that their needs may be reviewed in consultation with other practitioners with relevant expertise.

➤ Staff must ensure culturally appropriate ways of communicating that are courteous and clear and demonstrate a respect for privacy and dignity.

➤ Staff must respect the patient's right to choose whether to continue or withdraw: we may try to persuade, but ultimately this is the patient's/ clients own decision.

➤ Staff must understand issues of capacity and consent. Working with vulnerable people requires specific ethical awareness and competence. We must carefully consider issues concerning their capacity to give consent.

➤ Staff have a professional duty to respond to their clients' requests for information about the way that they are working and any assessment that they may have made. This professional requirement does not apply if it is considered that imparting this information would be detrimental to a client or inconsistent with the approach previously agreed with the client. Clients may have legal rights to this information, and these need to be taken into account.

➤ There must be no abuse of the client's trust in order to gain sexual, emotional, financial or any other kind of personal advantage. Practitioners should think carefully about, and exercise considerable caution before, entering into personal or business relationships with former clients, and should expect to be professionally accountable if the relationship becomes detrimental to the client or the standing of the profession.

➤ Practitioners must not allow their professional relationships with clients to be prejudiced by any personal views they may hold about lifestyle, gender, age, disability, race, sexual orientation, beliefs or culture.

➤ Practitioners should be clear about any commitment to be available to clients and colleagues, and honour these commitments.

➤ Conflicts of interest are best avoided, provided that they can be reasonably foreseen in the first instance and prevented from arising. In deciding how to respond to conflicts of interest, the protection of the client's interests and maintaining trust in the practitioner should be paramount.

3 Practitioners have a responsibility to protect clients from foreseeable harm
Practitioners must behave quickly and assertively if they have good reason to believe that a colleague is placing their client at risk of harm. They have a responsibility to raise any concerns with the colleague concerned in the first instance, unless it is inappropriate to do so. If the matter cannot be resolved, they should review the grounds for their concern and the evidence available to them and, when appropriate, raise their concerns with the practitioner's manager, agency or professional body. If the practitioner is uncertain what to do, their concerns should be discussed with an experienced colleague or a supervisor, or raised with their professional association, which will be able to advise on professional conduct procedures.

4 Practitioners have a responsibility to work in harmony with their colleagues
Professional relationships should be conducted in a spirit of mutual respect, and aim to maintain good working relationships and systems of communication that enhance services to clients at all times. For this, we need to be aware of some ground rules.

➤ All colleagues should be treated fairly and foster equality opportunity.

➤ We should not allow our professional relationships with colleagues to be prejudiced by our personal views about a colleague's lifestyle, gender, age, disability, race, sexual orientation, beliefs or culture. It is unacceptable and unethical to discriminate against colleagues on any of these grounds.

➤ We must not undermine a colleague's relationships with clients by making unjustified or unsustainable comments.

➤ All communications between colleagues about clients should be on a professional basis and thus purposeful, respectful and consistent with the management of confidences as declared to clients.

It would be wise for managers and supervisors of those in clinical practice to be aware of the types and extent of boundary violations that can occur. When an issue, the manager or supervisor needs to support their supervisee with their own reflections into what went wrong and why, and come to a better understanding of the above professional boundaries.

For further information about working with boundary issues, including some key examples of good and bad practice, *see* Chapter 14 of my sister book, *Developing Assertiveness Skills for Health and Social Care Professionals*.

The disciplinary interview is always perceived as challenging. It needs to be managed in such a way that both employer and employee feel safe and leave with a good outcome. Similar communication skills are required. Although these interpersonal and communication skills may look simplistic, they do need practise to perfect, and underpinning all of them is the ability to listen: carefully, calmly, actively, in a focussed way, without prejudice or judgement. The listener has to be assertive in their management of the situation, and ask questions, probe, reflect, accept criticism and summarise. They need to be seen to take charge, so the employee, patient or client feels that they are in safe hands, there is a boundary in place and something will happen as a result of the interview.

THE DISCIPLINARY INTERVIEW

The disciplinary interview is one of the most difficult events for both the manager and the member of staff, and because of this many managers avoid using the correct disciplinary procedures. Giving criticism is never easy, and if given badly it can lead to avoidable and expensive resignation. However, if one member of staff consistently makes mistakes and is not disciplined, the lack of boundaries and clarity can create a feeling of uncertainty among the other members of staff. They too may then work in an undisciplined way as they see the organisation condoning bad behaviour without sanction. Effective leaders create clear guidelines, limits and boundaries and are consistent and fair in their approach. They demonstrate that they understand the culture and model mutual respect and clarity. They clearly identify acceptable and unacceptable behaviour, and are not frightened to challenge unacceptable behaviour if it occurs.

We looked at giving and receiving criticism in Chapter 6 of my sister book, *Developing Assertiveness Skills for Health and Social Care Professionals*, but here we examine some of the communication skills needed to make workplace disciplining effective and easy.

Constructive criticism

The assertive person does not avoid expressing a grievance, and understands the negative effects of nursing grievances: it is always wiser to clear the air. We all need to be told when we are doing it wrong, in order that we may learn from the experience.

Criticism *is* difficult to confront. It does seem much easier to let resentment build up, as we may fear hurting someone, making a scene, creating the wrong impression or being disliked. Because badly given criticism can leave people feeling hurt or rejected, can feel like an attack, and can antagonise or confuse, we avoid giving criticism because we try to spare the pain. In this way, we protect people from their own feelings. But we do need to share our grievances before stored up resentments turn a small incident into a huge one. The aim is to communicate in a more civilised manner and face the problem directly. Communicating vague resentments is always passive and manipulative, and aggressive retorts leave people feeling hurt and angry, so if you feel angry and critical, stop and think: the only reason for giving criticism is to help the other person to grow, develop and learn from their mistakes. Allow people to accept or reject the criticism in their own way; they too are adults and must assume responsibility for dealing with the situation, and their feelings, as they wish. It is patronising to assume responsibility for your staff's emotional lives.

Giving constructive criticism
➤ Select your *time* and place wisely: use a private room and allow yourself ample time.
➤ Be *specific*. Do not drop vague hints that you are irritated by poor time keepers, confront the issue: 'Lynne, we feel frustrated when you are late – could you try to arrive by 4 o'clock next time?'
➤ Be *honest* and true to yourself, mean what you say.
➤ Be prepared to *compromise*: 'If this time is difficult for you, maybe we could think about starting the meeting later …'
➤ Take responsibility for, and express, your *feelings* about the behaviour, and the effect it has on you, the organisation or the patient/client: 'I feel uncomfortable when …'
➤ *Avoid judgement*, attack and blame – whether in the form of 'You're so immature' or 'You should be more …'. This can be read as unsolicited,

unwanted advice. Global or generalised statements about someone's behaviour are, basically, attacks on their personality. Again, state how you feel, specifically, about the one item of behaviour you want changed.

➤ Do not assume that you know what motivates other people, for you may be mistaken. *Avoid analysis* such as: 'You must have known how much that would hurt' – it is impossible to interpret other people's behaviour.

➤ Spell out the *consequences* of changed behaviour: 'I will feel much less strained if you could be on time.' If the change you anticipate or hope for does not come about, be prepared to ride the consequences. Remember that we can always change our behaviour, but we cannot expect others to change theirs, however much we want them too. You can ask, but you may not get what you want.

➤ View the other person as an *equal*. If you do take the initiative to confront, remember that you in turn may be confronted.

➤ If you have been avoiding raising the subject, take *responsibility*. Invariably, people are surprised, and often shocked, when you mention that part of their behaviour has had such an effect on you; so do take responsibility for not mentioning it before: 'I'm sorry that I didn't make myself clear before. I should have mentioned it, but I didn't feel able.'

➤ *Invite criticism*: 'Have I surprised/upset/angered you?'

➤ *Empathise*. Understand the other person's position. Start with something on the lines of: 'I realise that what I have to say will be upsetting …'

➤ Keep *calm*. Make sure that you keep your voice level and avoid using threatening gestures.

➤ *Phrase positively*. 'It would be better if you talked more loudly' gives someone the hope of being both better heard and better regarded if they make that change. Saying the same thing negatively, 'It would be better if you did not talk so quietly', can leave the person concentrating on their sense of failure rather than wanting to improve.

➤ *End on a positive note*. Find a remark to balance the interaction, give some indication that you value the other person and are not only seeing the negative: 'I'm grateful to you for listening' or 'I'm glad that we've aired this'. If you wish, you may like to add a positive statement about the other person: 'I do hope that my having said this will not adversely affect our relationship. I've always found you especially easy to talk to, and I do value the way we work so well together.' Or you may prefer to end the conversation with a positive consequence; something on the lines of: 'I'm glad that we've cleared the air. Now I feel that I'll be less tense during our meetings.'

The interview

Staff should be aware of any systems for discipline, and disciplinary procedures, in use. One of the reasons for having known policies, procedures, job descriptions and contracts is that staff will be aware when their work is not up to standard. It is then much easier to draw their attention to your expectations and the fact they have broken their side of the deal.

The objectives

The objective of a disciplinary interview is to inform of mistakes or unwanted behaviour and correct them by helping the employee to improve – thus preventing the situation from arising again. It should not be viewed primarily as a means of imposing sanctions.

Interviewing for disciplinary problems

Disciplinary problems are to do with people's performance: someone is not doing what he or she ought. The aim is to improve performance in the future. This means that the whole emphasis must be on the future, looking forward rather than back. The interview should be in a problem-solving style: getting the facts, exchanging opinions, deciding action. There are certain basic principles that will always apply to this kind of interview. You need to be seen to be taking the whole matter seriously. You need to listen and let the interviewee do much of the talking, as this is the only way to get the facts and co-operation, and to enable you fully to understand the problem. Keep calm and control your temper if you feel provoked: the aim is to solve a problem, and an aggressive attitude will never achieve this. You will need to focus on work performance, not personality. Finally, you need to aim for agreement on the problem and the action decided.

Specific techniques

Preparation

Ensure that the interviewee clearly understands that it is a disciplinary interview: that they have received a formal warning and that the interview may form part of a dismissal procedure. They should be told in advance that they have the right to be accompanied by someone else if they wish. Plan both the interview and the outcome in advance: you will aim for a successful outcome, which will almost certainly be a change of some kind in the employee's behaviour. Plan the interview:

➤ be clear about the reasons for seeing the employee
➤ have all the facts to hand
➤ try not to pre-judge
➤ plan your approach according to the individual
➤ consider your sanctions
➤ know the procedure inside out
➤ ensure privacy.

Opening

Indicate the context and measure of importance by making sure that you are seated: this is not a conversation to have informally. State the aim of the interview straight away, establish the objective: 'I want us to get to the bottom of this matter and agree what to do about it.' Be clear: 'I thought we'd better have a talk because of your timekeeping in the last few weeks.' Then, move on to ask the interviewee for their side of the story, and probe the information given. Did they know an offence was being committed? Investigate the facts of the case thoroughly through allowing the employee to put their case. Then, if the employee has not already identified his or her learning points, clarify the expected standards of performance or organisational policy. It is useful to begin and end on a positive note; if so, at this point, commend any good work and effort that you have noted.

Manner

Your manner throughout must be professional, calm, firm and fair. This is a serious matter; show that you are taking it seriously. Encourage frankness, and take care with your choice of words – the aim is not to patronise or humiliate.

Listen

Establish the facts. Do not get bogged down in recriminations about the past. Show you have been listening: summarise the employee's viewpoint and get them to agree that you have got it right. Ask open-ended questions that cannot be answered with just 'yes' or 'no' – 'What effect do you think this has on other people?'. Do not ask leading questions such as: 'When are you going to stop disrupting other people's work?' Having asked a question, wait for an answer – do not worry about pauses, and pay attention to everything said: try to detect the feelings and attitudes behind the words. Throughout, encourage talking with non-verbal encouragement: nods, smiles, 'Hmm', 'Yes, I see'.

Problem solving

Your aim is to reach agreement on what the problem is. Draw the employees' attention to the fact that their action has led to difficulties for their colleagues: this may have more impact than an explanation that you or the team has been let down – help them to understand your problem. Keep the discussion to the point. Be prepared to amend your original view, and encourage the employee to suggest solutions: discuss more than one possible solution. Make it clear that you cannot agree to grant any favours unless there are very special circumstances, and remind them of any known procedures, such as the next stages in an appeals procedure.

Conclusion

Agree on what you are both going to do and agree a time-scale for follow up.

Tell the employee whether you will be making any record of your interview or discussing the matter with anyone else, and check that you have achieved your immediate aims.

Follow up

Look for ways to help the employee avoid making the same mistake in the future, and decide on a reasonable length of time in which the employee must improve, then clarify that any action has been understood. Write up notes immediately. Take any action you agreed on to help the individual, sending copies to them, and fix a date to meet again.

Each disciplinary interview should be approached according to the stage of the procedure reached. Decide on the seriousness of the action. At the initial stages, an informal, problem-solving approach may be best, and considerate handling at this stage may prevent the matter from going any further.

In summary
➤ Discuss performance, not the person.
➤ Use facts, not assumptions.
➤ Be objective, use records.
➤ Spell out limits and aims.
➤ Listen.
➤ Share the blame, if necessary.
➤ Use mistakes to learn.
➤ Focus on the future, not the past.
➤ Find a better way.
➤ Affirm their ideas, compliment calm manners.
➤ Summarise.
➤ End on a high note.
➤ Follow up.

Problems in disciplinary interviews

The best approach for disciplinary interviews is the problem-solving approach. Sometimes, however, it seems to be the last approach the interviewee wants. If the interviewee tries to avoid the problem-solving approach, either by surrendering, attacking or avoiding, you should not be deflected. Be aware of and understand these tactics and know how to avoid them. In all the following examples,[8] keep to the main purpose of the interview, without being side-tracked.

➤ **The person who confesses everything.** They admit everything – including matters you did not intend to discuss. The aim is to deflect your aim from the one aspect you wanted to discuss.
  – *Action:* ignore the distractions, stick firmly to the point you want to discuss, for example: 'It's that time-keeping problem that I particularly want to discuss at the moment.'

➤ **The person who cries.** Hopes to embarrass the interviewer into backing down or abandoning the whole idea.
  – *Action:* offer tissues. Wait. Then gently – but firmly – proceed as planned.

➤ **The person who claims to be in deep depression and full of problems** – to which, hopefully, you will not add.
  – *Action:* if the depression is genuine, support external referral. If not, make it clear that you expect nothing exceptional – just the same standards as others and the same, presumably, as he or she formerly achieved.

➤ **The person who threatens their resignation.** An offer (threat?), usually accompanied by warnings of the difficulty of replacing him or her.
  – *Action:* be wary – accepting their offer could lead you into a 'constructive dismissal'. Stick to the topic of the interview, for example, 'We're not talking about resignation, we're trying to work out how to reduce the error rate on these reports.'

➤ **The 'ambusher'** who lies in wait, saying nothing until they have identified the weakness in your argument. Then they home in on it.
  – *Action:* be sure of your facts before you start. Ask questions to get them talking. If they do find a minor weakness, do not allow it to become the central issue, for example: 'The exact time does not affect the main issue – your being late three days out of five.'

➤ **The 'shop-steward'.** Usually knows the rule book inside out and claims also to speak on behalf of the 'department'.
  – *Action:* let them talk it out without being drawn into detailed arguments. Keep the focus on their behaviour, for example: 'Let's put on one side for the moment what the department thinks. What can you do to help solve this problem?'

➤ **The person who claims to be the injured, and innocent, party**, who cannot believe that they are being accused of doing something deliberately.

---

8   Fred Pryor Seminars. *Dealing with Difficult People*. Pryor Resources, Inc.; 1998.

- *Action:* ignore the emotive words they use. Do not start apologising for their deliberate misunderstanding of what you said: 'I just want to find out the reasons why the telephone was left unattended this morning.'

➤ **The buck passer** always has a hundred good reasons why it is not their fault: someone else let them down, etc.
  - *Action:* be sure of your facts before you start.

➤ **The aggressor** believes that attack is the best form of defence and will probably attack you verbally: your own work habits; your competence to discuss this with them, etc.
  - *Action:* do not lose your temper – that is what they want. Pin them down to what they are going to do towards solving the problem under discussion.

THE RESIGNATION, EXIT OR TERMINATION INTERVIEW

If your colleague feels threatened by the disciplinary procedure, he or she may react proactively by handing in their notice. If this occurs, listen carefully to their grievance as it can tell you some important facts about your organisation and style of management. It may be that the employee has had inadequate training for the job, or has been poorly supervised. It certainly points to unresolved problems or unvoiced grievances, which may mean that in future you need to be more aware of undercurrents of stress at work and need to allow space for these to be voiced.

Your objective is to discover the real reason for their wanting to resign, and then to use what you have learnt to prevent others from leaving. You may wish at this stage to persuade an individual to change his or her mind, but if you fail, wish them well in their choice as it is in your organisation's favour to secure employee goodwill.

FURTHER HELP

Always seek legal advice before embarking on a disciplinary procedure. Investigate all the training options before considering dismissal. You may need to seek the advice of:

➤ your line manager or senior management team

➤ your employing trust's human resources department

➤ your union, professional support organisation or industrial relations advisors

➤ the Advisory, Conciliation and Arbitration Service (see the ACAS Code of Practice on Disciplinary Practice and Procedures in Employment).

KEY POINTS

➤ The people and interpersonal communication skills needed in all types of interview are multifaceted, the skills required of the counsellor, negotiator, manager and organiser: good interpersonal, communication, problem-solving, analytical and planning skills.

➤ Good listening is hard, and requires high concentration and energy. Because of this, we, among other things, fake attention and we pre-judge – we hold prior expectations of what the speaker is about to say; our minds wander, and noise, distractions, time pressure and our own internal thoughts may interfere.

➤ The manager's role in most interviews is to clarify the reasons for the work-related difficulties before deciding on a course of action. The aim is not to tell but to help the interviewee to solve or come to terms with the problems themselves. The interviewer acts to provide a sense of choice and safety for the person being interviewed, with the manager providing a focus of evaluation, congruence, an open presence, encouragement and an ongoing commitment to the interviewee.

➤ The interviewee, if given adequate time and space with which to explore their problem, will know when the work begins and ends; but the manager commits to provide a safe boundary through agreeing some core conditions of time, frequency and confidentiality.

➤ The objective of a grievance interview is to enable the person to air a complaint, to discover the causes of dissatisfaction and, where possible, remove them. For this, prepare in advance, check your mutual understanding of the exact situation and the facts, probe deeply, and ensure that you both understand what happens next.

➤ Appraisals are another way of demonstrating that you believe in your staff. They can be viewed as a formal system for examining and building on your staff's strengths and minimising their weaknesses. The purpose is to work collaboratively jointly to review past performance, assess future potential, and find out what motivates and rewards the appraisee.

➤ In a clinical teaching role, you will be supporting, encouraging and developing your employee, colleague or student – clinically, professionally and personally. For this, we need to develop self-awareness, humility and constructive concern for the student's welfare.

➤ There are various formal and informal supervision models available, including buddy/mentor systems, peer support, clinical focus groups, professional case reviews, joint sessions, one to one with a senior practitioner or professional lead, and shadowing.

➤ In supervision, feedback should be goal related (towards clearly specified objectives) and timely (reducing feedback as the person progresses towards independence and competence).

➤ If one member of staff consistently makes mistakes and is not disciplined, the lack of boundaries and clarity can create a feeling of uncertainty among the other members of staff. They too then may work in an undisciplined way, as they see the organisation condoning bad behaviour without sanction.

➤ Effective leaders create clear guidelines, limits and boundaries and are consistent and fair in their approach. They demonstrate that they understand the culture and model mutual respect and clarity. They clearly identify acceptable and unacceptable behaviour, and are not frightened to challenge unacceptable behaviour if it occurs.

➤ The assertive person does not avoid expressing a grievance, and understands the negative effects of nursing grievances: it is always wiser to clear the air. We all need to be told when we are doing it wrong – in order that we may learn from the experience.

➤ Because badly given criticism can leave people feeling hurt or rejected, can feel like an attack, and can antagonise or confuse, we avoid giving criticism because we try to spare the pain. In this way, we protect people from their own feelings. The aim is to communicate in a more civilised manner and face the problem directly. Allow people to accept or reject the criticism in their own way – they too are adults and must assume responsibility for dealing with the situation, and their feelings, as they wish.

➤ When giving criticism, we must take care to keep calm, be specific, be honest, phrase positively, take responsibility for, and express, your feelings, avoid judgement and personal analysis, and treat the other person as an equal. Spell out the consequences of changed behaviour. You may need to invite criticism. Finally, be prepared to compromise and end on a positive note.

➤ The objective of a disciplinary interview is to inform of mistakes or unwanted behaviour and correct them by helping the employee to improve, thus preventing the situation from arising again. It should not be viewed primarily as a means of imposing sanctions.

In summary
➤ discuss performance, not the person
➤ use facts, not assumptions
➤ be objective, use records
➤ spell out limits and aims
➤ listen
➤ share the blame, if necessary
➤ use mistakes to learn
➤ focus on the future, not the past
➤ find a better way

> ➤ affirm their ideas, compliment calm manners
> ➤ summarise
> ➤ end on a high note
> ➤ follow up.

FURTHER READING

Bloch S, Kramer S, Parker A. Developing distance supervision. *Royal College of Speech and Language Therapists Bulletin.* 2010; **695**: 14–15.

Bruce C, Parker A, Herbert R. The development of a self-directed and peer-based clinical training programme. *International Journal of Language and Communication Disorders.* 2001; **36**: 401–415.

Gascoigne M, Parker A. All placements great and small: an analysis of clinical placement offers made by SLT services. *International Journal of Language and Communication Disorders.* 2001; **36**: 144–9.

Kersner M, Parker A. A strategic approach to clinical placement learning. *International Journal of Language and Communication Disorders.* 2001; **36**: 150–5.

Mearns D, Thorne B. *Person-centred Counselling in Action.* Counselling in Action series. 3rd ed. Sage Publications Ltd; 2007.

Parker A, Kersner M. Developing as a speech and language therapist. In: Kersner M, Wright JA, editors. *Speech and Language Therapy: the decision-making process when working with children.* David Fulton; 2001. pp. 12–29.

Parker A, Kersner M. New approaches to learning during clinical placement. *International Journal of Language and Communication Disorders.* 1998; **33**: 255–60.

Rogers C. *Client Centred Therapy: its current practice, implications and theory.* New edited ed. Constable; 2003.

Stevenson G, Parker A, Franklin S. *The Provision of Clinical Placements: stakeholder roles and responsibilities.* Royal College of Speech and Language Therapists; 2003.

CHAPTER 11

Delegating

The ability to delegate is a crucial skill for any worker to acquire. Clinical staff, chief executives, directors, managers, supervisors – all have a responsibility to delegate some of their work so that they can concentrate on those tasks that only they are best able, and paid, to do. It is very common among clinicians to find poor patterns of delegation: it is an underused art, and one that female practitioners in particular find hard. In this chapter, we look at why, how, when and what to delegate, and why some people find it so hard.

WHY DELEGATE?

➤ Good delegation gives you more time for thinking and planning – and taking the big decisions that cannot be delegated.
➤ The person closest to the activity should be better able to make decisions.
➤ Delegation tends to encourage initiative, which, in turn, improves morale.
➤ Delegation equips people to solve their own problems.
➤ Delegation reduces decision time.
➤ People enhance their contribution to the organisation by concentrating on tasks that they are best suited for.
➤ Good delegation makes you dispensable – and that should help your promotion chances.

WHY WE DO NOT DELEGATE

Although it is relatively easy to get people to agree that delegation is worthwhile, many do not delegate as effectively as they could. There are reasons for this – find which one below speaks to you.

➤ You manage your own time badly, you are overstretched and spend time doing instead of planning. This is one of the most common reasons for not delegating. Healthcare workers are working to capacity, but need to set aside time to think and plan to enable them to distinguish between the urgent things and the important things. Delegation leaves you free to give attention to more important matters.
➤ Your responsibilities and limit of authority are not clear to you, or anyone

else. If you are uncertain about your role, you simply cannot delegate effectively. Become certain. Find out.

➤ You underestimate the competence of your subordinates and genuinely believe that you can do the work better than anyone else. This is another common reason why women in particular do not delegate, at home and at work. It may be true, but it does not follow that you will get as much done as a properly co-ordinated work team. As we climb within our own hierarchy, the strategic content of the job increases as the operational, 'doing' content declines. We cannot hope to remain specialists with superior technical skills after moving into a job which has quite different requirements. Inadequate subordinates will never improve if you do their work for them. They must either be moved or developed (by delegation).

➤ You feel threatened by the competence of your subordinates. If this is the case, work to raise your self-esteem, and develop a more secure sense of self.

➤ You feel insecure in your job and in your work relationships. If so, and if delegation is the right to make decisions, then it must include the right to make mistakes, too, for anyone who makes decisions will inevitably make a mistake at some time. How big a mistake are you willing to let someone else make? Many managers fail to delegate because they fear the criticism if a mistake is made. However, to delegate properly, you must be confident that you can solve any problem which your subordinates may create, as to delegate is not to abdicate responsibility. Those who feel insecure in their positions make poor delegators for a variety of reasons. They may be afraid of not being essential; they may feel more competent and comfortable performing routine duties instead of the work of a manager – planning, organising, controlling, and leading; or they do not want to appear lazy – to their seniors, colleagues, and subordinates – or even to themselves.

Having identified the reasons why we tend to avoid delegating, let us examine some of the principles of delegation.

HOW TO DELEGATE

Delegation is the process by which a manager grants or permits the transfer of authority to someone to operate within prescribed limits. Whoever delegates has to have permission within the organisation to do so. Delegating is entrusting responsibility and authority to others (not necessarily subordinates), who then become responsible to you for results. The delegator remains accountable for the performance of their subordinates. What you delegate, essentially, is the right to make decisions. Authority and responsibility go hand in hand, as a person cannot be responsible for a task if authority to act is not given. Whoever delegates cannot avoid responsibility by delegation.

For delegation to be successful, the following needs to be in place.

It is imperative that everyone is clear about their role within the organisation, and for this the organisation needs to have clearly identified organisational objectives, policies and guidelines. It is important to have clear definitions of the responsibilities and authority of each job, in writing. This provides greater freedom than ambiguous or inconsistent boundaries.

There is no absolute rule as to the number that one person can effectively manage, as this depends on the nature of the work, the ability and training of your team, the degree of delegation, and the degree of communication distance. To summarise, delegation depends on who carries the following responsibilities.

➤ The *authority* to delegate: the person with the right and legitimate power to delegate responsibility.

➤ The *responsibility* to delegate involves an obligation by the subordinate to perform certain duties.

➤ *Accountability*: who carries ultimate responsibility.

To delegate well you need to be accessible, communicate with your subordinates, share thinking and objectives to provide a background for their decisions, inform them of your expectations and how results will be evaluated, and monitor the process. This follows various *stages*:

➤ the specific roles of both the delegator and those delegated to need to be outlined

➤ reasonable objectives need to be established and clarified

➤ terms of reference are to be agreed

➤ lines of authority and responsibility noted

➤ guidance, support and training offered

➤ agreement on any time schedule must be established, as must identification of specific results and means of measurement, monitoring and review periods.

The delegator trusts and permits the subordinate to act, allowing freedom of action within the agreed terms of reference, and finally notices a job well done by rewarding practically or with verbal praise. The person who has assumed responsibility for the task has a role to report back, so the person in charge can modify or recommend alternative action.

There is some debate about whether delegation should be seen as an art or a science. However it is viewed, good delegation does have some similarities with the application of an audit, which is cyclical in nature, has clearly identified and measurable aims and objectives, and is constantly reviewed and modified, depending on results. Thus delegators have a clear responsibility to communicate the aims and objectives of the job they are delegating.

Objectives should:

➤ be brief, yet cover the main features of the job

- be verifiable
- state the time by when they are to be achieved
- indicate the quality of objectives and the cost of achieving them
- present a challenge
- indicate priorities.

Good objectives indicate:
- quantity (how much)
- quality (how well, or specific characteristics)
- time (when)
- cost (at what cost).

Even if the objectives are qualitative in nature, they should still be expressed clearly, and be measurable and verifiable, and any priorities assigned to them should be able to be ranked or weighted. Objectives set should be challenging, yet reasonable. They need to be communicated to all who need to be informed. Are the objectives co-ordinated with other departments? Are they consistent with the objectives of the organisation, with any underlying assumptions clearly identified? A good delegator will ensure that the objectives provide timely feedback so that any necessary corrective steps can be taken, and that the resources and authority given are sufficient for achieving the objectives.

If using delegation as a means of developing subordinates, review the situation regularly and discuss overall performance. In this review, consider how well the agreed objectives have been achieved and what could be done to improve. Suggest suitable objectives for the next period, and ways in which the job might change in the future. In this interview, listen to the subordinate's views on the problems encountered in working towards their objectives: whether they now think the objectives were unrealistic; ways in which you could have helped more; ways in which they think the job has changed; and where they want to go from here. Agree on what the next job is, and what you are trying to achieve, then agree on what you are each going to do to meet that objective. Use this interview to establish whether the individuals who are expected to accomplish objectives were given a chance to suggest their own, and if they had sufficient control over aspects for which they were assigned responsibility.

EXERCISE 1

Which bird of delegation are you?[1]

- **The white-shirted hoverer:** a bird that gives a subordinate a job to do and then perches on their shoulder.

---

1   Source: Supervisor's pack. Brighton College of Technology; 1997.

➤ **The pin-striped whoopster:** a bird that watches closely over its subordinates and becomes very raucous when they deviate from the way it thinks the job should be done.

➤ **The yellow-bellied credit snatcher:** a bird well known and often highly regarded.

➤ **The lesser white-crested cuckoo:** the bird that, by habit, lays its eggs in another's nest.

➤ **The duck-billed double-talker:** a bird that really never made clear what authority it meant to delegate.

➤ **The golden-crowned mourning dope:** a bird that mourns the lack of people it can trust with decisions, yet that will not let anyone else decide anything.

➤ **The black and white organisation creeper:** the bird that delegates authority and then creeps around the structure to lower-level subordinates and thereby nullifies the delegation.

➤ **The redheaded firefighter:** the bird that thinks it is delegating authority when it asks its subordinates to check with it before making even the most minor decisions.

➤ **The lion-kicking vulture:** sits back and waits for its subordinates to make important mistakes and then kicks these 'dead lions' with gusto and bravado.

WHEN, WHAT AND WHAT NOT TO DELEGATE

Let your own subordinates control their work, even if they do not handle things quite as well as you to begin with. Remember that each job should be tackled at the lowest possible level. Delegate as a contribution to staff training and development. If you feel you cannot trust a subordinate with a job, train them. It is useful to delegate to assess suitability for promotion.

In general, the subordinate should tackle predictable tasks, while the more experienced should handle exceptional ones. These types of task should be delegated down:

➤ matters that keep repeating themselves
➤ minor decisions most frequently made
➤ details that take the biggest chunks of time
➤ parts of the job the delegator is least qualified to handle
➤ job details the superior most dislikes
➤ parts of the job that make the superior overspecialised.

Leaders should not delegate any key management roles – the things that only they can do such as overall policy decisions, planning, selection, training and appraisal, promotion, praise and disciplinary action of immediate subordinates, or final accountability for the work of their department. Setting objectives is the responsibility of management, as is organising employees into an efficient team, motivation, communication, and control functions such as checking and analysing results. The manager needs to take full responsibility also for confidential matters, legally or contractually restricted jobs. For these the manager assumes ultimate accountability. Generally, delegators should not delegate anything to people who are not capable of doing the work effectively, or to people who do not work for them.

In summary, to delegate:

Anything someone can do *better*, *quicker*, *cheaper* than or *instead* of, you.

EXERCISE 2

Consider whether you delegate fairly and competently and have planned for your succession.

➤ Draw up a list of the job responsibilities you would leave behind if you were suddenly to leave your practice.

➤ List the subordinates qualified to take over each of those responsibilities. If there is no one available, leave a blank.

➤ Give each blank one of the following reasons:
  – inadequate subordinate (for whatever reason)
  – poorly defined management structure
  – your choice (for whatever reason).

➤ Make a list of the duties which you could delegate but do not. Work out why you do not.

➤ Make a list of duties that could be delegated to you. Establish why this has not happened.

Making it easier to delegate

Be sure that you and your boss agree on what your job is, and be sure that your subordinates understand what you expect them to do: agree their area of responsibility and the required standards of performance, then give them the means of carrying out their task: authority, knowledge, materials, people and, preferably, a budget. Specify objectives in qualitative terms, with a target date for completion – but allow your subordinate to choose their own methods, let them take their own decisions, with guidance whenever requested, subject to periodic checks and feedback. Build up confidence by resisting the desire to over-criticise if a mistake is made. Discourage subordinates from 'half-taking' decisions and leaving the rest to you – get them to think problems right through and to act on their judgement, while ensuring that you set up a control system so that you can correct deviations from agreed standards. Reward the people who get things done. People will accept responsibility and actively participate in accomplishing the objectives of the organisation only if they feel that the rewards go to the people who get things done. The rewards for being right must always be greater than the penalties for being wrong. These rewards will include knowledge of results and, in a non-recession climate, promotion, pay – otherwise a friendly chat, respect and so on.

If you are having some problems with delegation,[2] ask questions, check that you are not taking advantage of key people who have more knowledge and experience than you in certain aspects of the work, and that you are not overloading high achievers. Check that you are not taking advantage simply in terms of time (because they are on the spot) or salary costs (because they are paid less). If so, try rotating jobs, or stop delegating and use the mistakes made for learning. The less than ideal solution at the right time may be far better than the otherwise ideal solution at the wrong time.

EXERCISE 3

How well do you delegate?

➤ Are decisions in your organisation made at the lowest level at which they can properly be made?
➤ Do your subordinates know what you expect them to do?
➤ Do your subordinates have policies to guide them in making decisions?
➤ Is your department organised in a way that facilitates delegation?
➤ Do you direct your subordinates to accomplish certain results, or simply to perform certain activities?
➤ Do you make the fullest possible use of your staff?
➤ Do you spend enough time on the really important parts of your job?
➤ Do you spend too much time 'putting out fires' – dealing with constant emergencies demanding your personal attention, which keep you from working on the major issues?
➤ Does your work face constant deadline crises, with some dates missed and others only just 'getting under the wire'?
➤ Do you regularly take work home or stay late in the office?
➤ Do you yield to the temptation to take your coat off and do the job yourself?
➤ Ask yourself: 'What should I be doing and what should I not be doing?'
➤ Ask yourself: 'How can I best equip each of my subordinates to do what they should be doing?'

---

2   Fred Pryor Seminars. *Delegation Dilemmas*. Pryor Resources, Inc.; 1997.

EXERCISE 4

Find out your areas of strength and weakness

Score your performance out of ten for each item, then get members of your staff and your senior to score you for a selection of the items. They may see things differently.

Question		Rating		
		Self	*Staff*	*Senior*
1	How much freedom of action do you allow your subordinates?			
2	Are you under pressure, unable to keep on top of the job?			
3	Do you keep subordinates informed about company policies?			
4	Do you adequately communicate the facts of changing situations to enable your subordinates to make good decisions?			
5	Is your superior prepared to encourage you to delegate by giving you added responsibility?			
6	Are you sufficiently courageous to risk subordinates making a mistake when it is you who may have to take the rap?			
7	Are you prepared to let others have a go, even if they do not do it your way?			
8	Your subordinates do the technical, routine and repetitive tasks: do you also give them the opportunity to be creative?			
9	Do you encourage subordinates to set their own work targets?			
10	Is it possible for your staff to monitor their own work progress?			
11	Are you subordinates encouraged to learn new skills or to improve their existing skills?			
12	Are your subordinates encouraged to take greater responsibility for their own work?			
13	Do you recognise the importance of delegating only within the range of competence of the individual?			

Question	Rating		
	Self	Staff	Senior
14 Do you accept your responsibility to develop subordinates to take on greater responsibility, and do you act on it?			
15 Have you systematically identified the activities you wish to delegate in the interest of motivating your subordinates as well as your own time-effectiveness?			
16 Do you monitor the delegated task and give positive feedback on how it is being performed?			
17 Do you accept that you remain accountable for all delegated activities?			
18 Do you delegate some tasks simply because you dislike them?			
19 Do you resist delegating some tasks because you enjoy them?			
20 Do you properly reserve to yourself or colleagues all decisions on policy?			
21 Have the responsibilities of your subordinates been clarified and communicated by means of detailed job descriptions?			
22 Are individuals made aware of their opportunities for growth and development by means of regular performance appraisals?			
23 Do you delegate the right to be wrong?			
24 When dealing with questions, do you ask the individual how he or she would handle it?			
25 Do you analyse bad decisions and learn from them?			

EXERCISE 5

Consider which of these tasks are managing the job and which are actually doing the job.[3]

1 *Calling a meeting to gain information from staff on how quality could be improved.* This is managing – but ask an assistant to arrange meeting venue/ times.

---

3 Fred Pryor Seminars, note 2 above.

2 *Reviewing appraisal records.* This is managing, as it is handling confidential information.

3 *Signing an authorisation form for routine stationary restocking.* This can be delegated – get someone else to sign up to a certain limit.

4 *Lunching with a visitor from outside the organisation who is touring your facilities.* This may be considered both managing and doing: it is a public relations exercise that could be given to someone in order to develop them, but it depends on who the visitor is.

5 *Working up a new system for decreasing nursing supplies.* Not managing, but doing.

6 *Calling former job references to verify employment dates.* A job to delegate.

7 *Attending a routine but important meeting on recent guidelines on reimbursement.* Delegate: ask one of your staff to go for you and report back.

KEY POINTS

➤ The ability to delegate is a crucial skill to acquire for any worker. We all have a responsibility to delegate some of our work so that we can concentrate on those tasks that only we are best able, and paid, to do.

➤ Although it is relatively easy to get people to agree that delegation is worthwhile, many do not delegate as effectively as they could. There are reasons for this: poor time management, unclear lines of responsibility, under- or overestimation of subordinates, and job insecurity.

➤ It is imperative that everyone is clear about their role within the organisation, and for this the organisation needs to have clearly identified organisational objectives, policies and guidelines.

➤ In delegating, think about who carries the authority, the responsibility and the ultimate accountability in the procedure.

➤ To delegate well, you need to be accessible, communicate with your subordinates, share thinking and objectives to provide a background for their decisions, inform them of your expectations and how results will be evaluated, and monitor the process.

➤ Even if the objectives are qualitative in nature, they should still be expressed clearly, and be measurable and verifiable, and any priorities assigned to them should be able to be ranked or weighted. Objectives set should be challenging, yet reasonable. They should be communicated to all who need to be informed.

➤ Let your own subordinates control their work, even if they do not handle things quite as well as you to begin with. Remember that each job should be tackled at the lowest possible level. In general, the subordinate should tackle predictable tasks, while the more experienced should handle exceptional ones.

➤ The manager needs to take full responsibility for confidential matters – legally or contractually restricted jobs, for which the manager assumes ultimate accountability.

➤ In delegating, you agree the area of the subordinate's responsibility and the required standards of performance, then give them the authority, knowledge, materials, people and a budget.

➤ Specify objectives and a target date for completion, letting people make their own decisions, with guidance whenever requested, subject to periodic checks and feedback.

➤ People will accept responsibility and actively participate in accomplishing the objectives of the organisation only if they feel that the rewards go to the people who get things done.

> ➤ Delegate anything someone can do *better, quicker, cheaper* than or *instead* of, you.

FURTHER READING

Genett D. *If You Want it Done Right, You Don't Have to Do it Yourself: the power of effective delegation*. Quill Driver Books; 2004.

Harvard Business School Press. *Delegating Work: expert solutions to everyday challenges*. Harvard Pocket Mentor Series. Harvard Business School Press; 2008.

Luecke R, Mcintosh P. *The Busy Manager's Guide to Delegation*. Worksmart Series. Amacom; 2009.

Mullins LJ. *Management and Organisational Behaviour*. 8th ed. Financial Times/Prentice Hall; 2007.

Smart JK. *Real Delegation: how to get people to do things for you – and do them well*. Prentice Hall; 2002.

Section 4

Applying leadership skills

CHAPTER 12

Personal development

Personal development covers any activity that improves awareness and identity, develops talents and potential, builds human skill and facilitates employability, enhances quality of life and contributes to the realisation of aspirations. The concept is not limited to self-help, but includes formal and informal activities for developing others, in roles such as teacher, guide, counsellor, manager, coach or mentor. In the context of the workplace, it refers to the methods and systems that support employee development at an individual level,[1] and may include:

➤ improving self-awareness and self-knowledge
➤ building or renewing personal identity
➤ developing strengths and talents
➤ spiritual development
➤ identifying or improving potential and thus building employability
➤ enhancing quality of life
➤ improving health and personal autonomy
➤ fulfilling aspirations
➤ defining and executing personal development plans
➤ improving social skills.

Personal development is also about establishing identity, developing competence, purpose and integrity, and mature interpersonal relationships; managing emotions; and achieving autonomy and interdependence.[2]

In previous chapters, we have looked at improving self-awareness, self-knowledge and interpersonal communication skills. This final section explores some of the ways by which it is possible to continue with self-development, fulfil aspirations, improve health and personal autonomy, and help improve employability through applying some of these developed skills to:

➤ develop relationships within your organisation
➤ manage your own time and stress levels

---

1 Aubrey B. *Managing Your Aspirations: developing personal enterprise in the global workplace.* McGraw-Hill; 2010. p. 9.
2 Chickering A, Reisser L. *Education and Identity.* Jossey-Bass; 1993.

➤ set goals and manage change
➤ use personal development plans.

The concept of personal development covers a wider field than self-development or self-help: personal development also includes developing other people. This may take place through roles such as those of teacher or mentor, either through a personal competency (such as the skill of certain managers in developing the potential of employees) or a professional service (such as providing training, assessment or coaching). Within organisations, personal development can occur through either the provision of employee benefits or the fostering of development strategies. Employee benefits can enhance both employers and employees by improving satisfaction, motivation, loyalty, productivity, innovation and quality. Employee surveys help organisations to find out personal development needs, preferences and problems, and they use the results to redesign parts of their organisation. The NHS, for example, as a large and forward-thinking public sector employer, usually offers training programmes as well, which help to support employee development, such as time and stress management, counselling, career development, assertiveness, managing conflict, teamwork and competency development. Personal development also forms an element in self-assessment tools, such as assessing one's level of ability using a competency grid, feedback from a 360-degree questionnaire or from external sources, such as patients/clients or other interested stakeholders.

This last section explores your own personal development, and:
➤ how you can apply assertiveness skills to develop yourself and your relationships at work
➤ some of the behaviours of good and bad managers
➤ some of the skills you may need to acquire if you are seeking promotion
➤ those skills you need to develop to gain more respect for your present abilities
➤ those skills required to manage your boss and colleagues more effectively.

If you know yourself better, you are more likely to be able to take control of your life, and live it actively rather than passively. As you take on more responsibility, a different kind of respect is demanded, which has both financial and personal implications. Those unused to this new role may need to learn new personal skills to support their new sense of self.

MOVING ON AND UP
➤ Does your work provide you with opportunities for growth and learning?
➤ Will you get bored with what you are doing in the next five years, or 15?

➤ Are the salaries at your job level sufficient for you to be able to provide for both your present and future financial needs?

➤ How much authority to make decisions do you have?

➤ Does your job adversely influence your home life?

➤ Do you feel that you are making a worthwhile contribution through your work?

Doing good work at the moment will get you recognised, but it may not be enough to get you promoted, because jobs at different levels call for very different qualities and skills. You may be intelligent, competent and skilled at what you do, but you may need to consider what your team leader or manager does that you do not. Put aside your own prejudices. It is simplistic to think that managers waste time on the phone all day long, talking to their friends, as the friends may be crucial connections who are vital to the job. To develop at work, you need to:

➤ network, build relationships

➤ join professional organisations and take an active role in them

➤ use every phone conversation and every meeting as a chance to make contacts

➤ take the time to talk with people so that vital relationships can grow

➤ learn from these connections and pass information on to your manager

➤ introduce your manager to important connections.

If you are seeking promotion, convince your employer that you have the higher-level capabilities that it is looking for – people do not risk on unproven quantity. To do so, you need to analyse the job for which you are aiming, look at what the people at that level are doing, and locate the key qualities and skills required.

If you think you are not being promoted because your manager will not acknowledge how you have changed, you have not changed in a way that is essential for success at the next level. If you feel you are seen in 'the same old way', consider the following.

➤ How do you think your organisation views you at work?

➤ What kind of person does it promote?

➤ What are the qualities in these people? Enthusiasm? Confidence? Ability to motivate?

➤ Do they see that you have the necessary qualities for promotion?

➤ Make a list of your possible weaknesses and analyse them.

➤ Do any of your weaknesses present major handicaps at the next level?

Once you have determined what characteristic might be holding you back, decide whether you value the quality, or if you want to change.

Never accept more responsibility without the corresponding job title. In the current political climate, when there is less money and organisations have a 'flatter' organisational structure with less opportunity for promotion, it is common for people to be asked to take on roles more suitable for those in a more senior position, or to be a 'champion' in a field of work – an unpaid expert. Before you agree to this, consider your position carefully. Do you need the experience? How will this benefit you as well as the organisation? If resources constrain, it may not be that you are being exploited, but that there are limited opportunities to do challenging work. However, if for you the reward of flattery or experience is not enough, and negotiating a pay rise or promotion is out of the question, politely decline. But if circumstances and resources permit, you are entitled to have the title to match what you are doing so that your responsibilities are clear to people, both internally and externally. Your employer's negotiating strength is based on giving you the opportunity you want so badly; your strength is behaving as if you are a gift to them: they want you to do the new work. And it is not easy to replace someone who already understands the organisation: it is time-consuming, costly and risky.

Promotion within the same organisation

Once you have been newly promoted, your working methods will need to change, as taking on a new management position will result in the development of new loyalties. Previously, the organisation may have been considered in terms of what it could do for you. You now need to address what is good for the organisation, for your staff and for yourself. Your job subtly changes: the things you used to do are taken out of your hands, the working relationships change. You will be learning the new job while you are training others into your old job. You will have the opportunity to redefine your creativity within a wider framework. You can still do the work better than most people, only now you can tell others how to do it better as well.

The way you first approach your new staff will make the difference between whether you will be effective as a leader or not. There are several diplomatic basics that a manager must bear in mind if he or she wants to be successful at it, and they are essential to doing the job.

Tips for the new manager

➤ First, assert the fact that you are the new leader/manager.
➤ Present yourself as a new person, welcoming the people who are already there.
➤ Set a cordial, formal friendliness at the start: but do not isolate yourself: you need to develop relationships and insights into the way people think.

> First, identify with and relate to your peers – it may be nice to have the post room people on your side, but they have to deliver your mail whether you expend a lot of energy on them or not.
> Remember, you represent your title as well as yourself, and do not be afraid to use the clout of that title to demand a certain respect.

If managing friends:
> acknowledge and discuss the difficulties with them honestly
> try to get a pledge of commitment to work towards a positive goal
> consider how others may view the friendship
> be alert to taking out frustrations on friends – you both know each other's weaknesses.

If managing older/more experienced colleagues:
> tap into their experience and knowledge of the organisation
> try for a pledge of non-competition
> their age and length of service equals commitment – get them involved
> seek out their assistance when training/mentoring new staff.

Being liked is not a key to functioning well in the job. It is much more important to engender a sense of respect for yourself as a professional. If you are seen as too friendly, staff will take up too much of your time. Provide a place where your people can work and express their talents to the full, and you will be considered a good leader. The need for acceptance is a powerful factor in the human psychology, as is the fear of rejection. When you compliment someone who works for you, you are using a powerful tool in building loyalties and improving motivation. When you comment negatively on an employee's work, you are playing on their fear of rejection. Under such psychological pressure, people are not able to perform at their best, and may seek to undermine your position. Try to limit threats to whip staff into line – people respond better to positive tactics. Create a situation where people want to come to work: you will have fewer problems with resentments, fewer demands for pay increases and fewer complaints about conditions.

Act with competence and instil a sense of being in charge by handling the problems that come your way: if your staff trust you, they will feel more comfortable and more motivated to do their best. If you have quirks, make them predictable personality traits and not sudden demonstrations of irrational behaviour. Your staff must believe that you are capable of doing your job, since how you do it affects how they do theirs. Do not create scenes: especially over the working habits of people who are working well overall. It outrages them, spoils their focus, wrecks their enthusiasm and destroys your own credibility.

WHAT SKILLS CONSTITUTE A GOOD MANAGER?

If you question colleagues about what makes a good manager, they will often cite valued personal qualities: kindness, humour, respect, good listening skills. Intuitively, we see the best management skills as people skills – empathy, foresight, flexibility, generosity and tolerance – along with problem-solving ability, organisational and assertiveness skills. In seeking to mature into a good, competent and valued manager, these skills are required, and those seeking management or leadership positions would be wise to skill up.

Experience suggests that it is good to develop *problem-solving* skills, where you devise a technique to arrive at solutions. If the problem involves a direct work situation, make a decision based on your experience. If not, use other people's experience to assist: discuss problems and their solutions collectively. Your forte is to be able to recognise the solution and 'decide' on it; you do not have to have the answers – just the ability to find them. If a problem develops, it now becomes your job to find out whether the system is at fault or the people. Your job will be to ask and listen: those doing the job are best qualified to tell you where the inefficiencies are. Be assertive and act: never ignore problems that do not seem to be your province; if there are unclear and unspoken resentments about co-workers and efficiency is affected, take appropriate steps.

Good managers *delegate responsibly* – work completed as scheduled demonstrates whether staff are working efficiently – but never make unreasonable demands around a deadline. Make it clear that you understand that circumstances, not just incompetence or stupidity, cause delays: people who work under conditions free from blame make fewer mistakes. If *mistakes* are made, point them out and allow for an explanation. Accept certain mistakes as inevitable; look for a solution together.

Be *flexible*, maintain a sense of the outside world and create a real understanding of a home/life balance. If employees are producing and achieving well, and the outcomes set for them are being met, you do not need to worry so much about formalities such as 9 to 5 punctuality if this is not essential to their work. They are working for you, and for themselves, too. Accept that some staff are using their job as a stepping-stone to another job – perhaps yours – and that your own position is ultimately a temporary one.

Part of your role will be offering *financial support* along with practical and emotional support. You may need to determine that an employee deserves a rise – and to handle the situation when this cannot be granted. As a manager, you sit between organisational policy and employees' needs. You cannot be a revolutionary and ruin your reputation with management, and you cannot alienate your staff by taking a hard line: present a fair and urgent appeal when there is a real need to get more money for staff. Always keep people informed of your efforts, and if you cannot ask for a rise at a particular time, be straightforward about it, providing honest suggestions if necessary.

Formal and informal *meetings* are the best way to gather ideas from the people most able to advise: make sure your staff see their value. A frequent exchange of ideas will help staff to view one another's talents and maintain your position as the final authority. Emphasise the importance of meetings by the times you schedule them, and expect people to be punctual.

If you have to make *uncomfortable decisions*, do not allow guilt to invade the issue. It only places you in a vulnerable position and you may make concessions you will regret. Actions such as firing, reprimanding or refusing rises do create emotional pressure and should be approached with the correct intent – that of maintaining the function and efficiency of your department. They should not be emotional decisions. Accept that hiring and firing people is part of being a boss. Do not moralise or try to justify your actions, but keep accurate documentation of the incidents that led you to your decision. Do not give ground if challenged, and remember that you have the right to demand competence from your staff.

Weak managers undermine and invalidate their staff. There is no room in any organisation for managers who make subtle derogatory remarks that *undercut self-confidence* instead of helping the person gain an awareness of their talents. Talented people will be more willing to work for those who appreciate them: you will get better results and more recognition. Managers who *threaten or bully* reveal their own insecurities. People are not so scared that they cannot see through such a ploy. Such behaviour is unacceptable. Staff should be a unit of various ideas, plans, dreams and talents. A manager has the responsibility not only for making final decisions, but also for utilising the talents that they are being paid for. Find the merits in ideas and requests, and when you must refuse something, do it with encouragement to continue generating new ideas. Poor managers are *timid*. Either they do not trust their own judgement or they are afraid of being disliked. There is no place in business for a manager who cannot say 'no'. Saying 'no' does not stifle talents and creativity, and if you do not take charge staff may gain so much ascendancy that they start to dictate what should be your prerogatives.

Be assertive:

➤ do not avoid difficult situations or accept mediocrity
➤ face your insecurities, and learn how to cope with authority
➤ listen, ask questions, take advice and then act
➤ allow yourself to make mistakes – assurance will come with experience
➤ remember that there is no such thing as the perfect boss
➤ bring yourself into the best focus possible
➤ remember that good intentions are as important as any other quality
➤ you have the responsibility to use all your capabilities.

PLAN YOUR OWN CAREER

It is said that in life there are four types of people:

➤ *people who watch things happen*
➤ *people to whom things happen*
➤ *people who do not know what is happening*
➤ *people who make things happen.*

If you are concerned for your future, or feel that your work is limiting you, give yourself some time to reflect and answer the following questions, developed by McGill and Beaty.[3]

EXERCISE 1

Who: mentally scan all the people who may be relevant to you, and what you may need to do to develop this network.
What: are the key areas you can tackle quickly to provide early success.
Where: reflect on your work and living environment.
When: timing is crucial. You need to be in the right place at the right time – when to act or not act is a highly developed skill.
How: think about new, creative and innovative actions. Trust your intuition. The behaviour that caused the problem is unlikely to solve it.
Why: think about your personal, professional and organisational needs.

Personal

➤ Do you pay sufficient attention to your personal needs?
➤ What support is available and do you use it well?
➤ What work pressures do you inflict on yourself and your family?
➤ How does your work enhance or detract from the quality of your life?
➤ Who controls how you use your time?

Professional

➤ Do you prefer to lead or be lead?
➤ Do you prefer stability or initiating change?
➤ Do you know, or want to know, how others perceive you? How can you find out?

Organisational

➤ What recent changes are affecting you the most and how?
➤ In which areas of work do you feel most comfortable and most uncomfortable?

---

3   McGill I, Beaty L. *Action Learning: a practitioner's guide.* Revised 2nd ed. Routledge; 2001.

➤ Why are you working in health services and what would make you want to leave?
➤ What opportunities does the health sector offer you as a career? What are the expectations and constraints?
➤ How has your job changed over the past year?
➤ What did you achieve?
➤ What would you like to do more of?
➤ What does your past performance tell you about your strengths, weaknesses, and needs for training and development?
➤ What type of work would you ideally like to do?
➤ What are the key conditions you require to provide you with job satisfaction?

EXERCISE 2

From answering these questions, what changes do you need to make?

To impress potential employers, you need to be able to demonstrate certain key skills that will enhance your personal effectiveness, can be learned and demonstrated, will improve your employability and help enable you to move between jobs, perhaps even between the public and private sectors. It will be increasingly important for healthcare workers to demonstrate that they can take on any developmental and strategic work needed in their organisation. Through your present job, you can demonstrate your ability to think analytically, and show how you manage your time and prioritise your work. Employers especially value the following skills:

➤ assertiveness, communication
➤ numeracy
➤ use of information technology
➤ continually improving one's own learning and performance.

Others cite ability to work with others and problem solving. The Association of Graduate Recruiters cites the following skills most in demand, in order of priority.[4] Mark off those that you already have, or can aspire to:

➤ team working
➤ interpersonal skills
➤ motivation
➤ enthusiasm
➤ flexibility
➤ customer awareness
➤ business awareness

---

4 www.agr.org.uk (accessed April 2013).

➤ problem solving
➤ planning and organisation.

Take the time now to reflect on the skills that you have now, both in paid work and any other area of your life. At interview, you may need to demonstrate how, in your present job, you:

➤ co-operate with your fellow workers (team working)
➤ seek and build relationships with colleagues (networking)
➤ listen to and consider a range of opinions, explain alternatives and make recommendations (organisational skills and flexibility)
➤ handle complaints, interview and appraise staff, chair meetings (interpersonal communication skills)
➤ manage finances (numeracy)
➤ use information technology
➤ develop customer awareness (promotion of a patient survey/participation group, or set up a proactive complaints procedure)
➤ plan and develop services.

In job applications, use language that accurately reflects your personal communication style so that your future employer can see whether your face fits, and draw attention to other key sought-after personal qualities such as honesty, reliability and sensitivity. If you are an organiser with an eye on the future, someone who sees the big picture rather than the detail, use language which indicates completion of a goal: active verbs (ending in -*ing*: organis*ing*, forward plann*ing*, problem solv*ing*). This demonstrates positivism, motivation and enthusiasm. It demonstrates the ability to plan ahead, problem solve and think strategically. Passive verbs demonstrate your steadfastness and staying power: these verb endings indicate solidity and reliability on your CV and at interview: 'I plan services, organise the appointment systems, solve problems as they present' – this indicates you feel more comfortable dealing with present crises rather than anticipating, planning and strategising.

Most employers in the (primarily bureaucratic) public sector are still looking for good planning and organisational skills – creativity and imagination are not commonly requested attributes. Entrepreneurs and opportunists are not generally sought after, but may be needed to complement teams. GPs, for example, may need to seek a complement to their individualism, as general practice tends to attract clinicians who prefer to work alone, or entrepreneurs – it may be advisable for those who recruit to balance these traits.

There are other skills that you can develop in your quest for promotion. Plan, prioritise, set standards for yourself and better them. If you want to succeed you need to manage your superiors as well as yourself. First, you will need to build a good relationship with your own manager.

MANAGING YOUR MANAGER

This relationship is critical because of the power your employer holds over you. You therefore need both to manage yourself and to develop the relationship you have with your manager. Your manager may cause you problems and sometimes the greatest anxiety, but he or she can also be a mentor, giving you a wider view of the world. It is important to understand their world, values and problems. Your boss reports to someone just as you do, even chairs and chief executive officers report to the board of directors, and ultimately to any shareholders and the public.

People succeed when they are motivated to work hard at something that singled them out. Without ambition there is little progress. However, more people have failed at work through not being able to fit in or establish good relationships on the job than for any other reason. Relationships, and good communication, are of the essence. Be strategic in developing important working relationships and this will put you in good stead when moving on and up. Understand your manager's responsibilities. Find out who they report to: it will help to know what pressures and demands are put on them. Understand what your boss is dependent on you for: if you can help your manager to function well, you may make a powerful ally. See the relationship for what it is without the emotional overtones, then your ego will not be destroyed every time you are asked to do something you may not want to do. It will help if you deal with your manager with the same care and objectivity that you deal with associates and subordinates: be a friend within the bounds of the relationship. Maintain communication: inform your manager of any problems, so that they are not surprised or unprepared for any consequences, but do not waste time relating trivial or non-essential matters.

Learn to qualify and quantify your productivity. Assess yourself and so increase your efficiency and effectiveness. Look at the cost of your work: the quantity, the quality and the time it takes to produce a certain amount of work. Quantify and share your value to the organisation using measurable factors such as the number of enquiries, presentations or complaints, or the amount of income or profit generated through your activities. To help you with your personal or career development, you may wish to take outside work, but first check that there is no conflict of interests and whether you need authority for a special dispensation. There may be an organisational policy carrying restrictions to doing other work. Be loyal. It is important to your integrity and to the trust placed in you.

Have frequent meetings with your boss. It is not enough to have performance reviews once a year. A request for more frequent meetings is legitimate and shows your concern beyond the immediate task to be done; it demonstrates an attempt to understand the thinking and planning of upper management. Use the meeting to:

➤ check you are meeting objectives
➤ understand required standards of performance
➤ gain useful information about the needs of the organisation
➤ update your boss with information
➤ gain feedback so to improve your performance
➤ confront difficult situations, and solve problems, together.

The manager who fails you

You have to decide when it is possible, practical and politic to use your superior to help to solve a work problem and when to turn elsewhere. Then you will not be victimised by the real, or imagined, failings of your manager. Here are some circumstances, noted by Dickson,[5] when you may feel failed by your manager, and some considered ways of managing the situation assertively.

If you feel that your manager no longer listens or communicates well and is no longer *accessible*, you may feel overlooked and ignored. Consider that you may have disappointed or dissatisfied your manager and he or she has unassertively begun to withdraw their attention. Here they are not being assertive, so you have to take the lead and solicit constructive criticism – ask: identify the problem. Are you creating extra work for your manager in some way? Are you asking too many questions but not providing the recommendations, opinion or judgement required? Take charge and offer solutions: 'Here's what I think we should do …' instead of 'What should I do?'. Offer solutions to problems that have arisen while you are doing the assigned work, thus exercising your own initiative. It may strengthen your relationship with your boss and give you an edge when being considered for promotion. Never ask your manager for information you can get from others. By keeping informed through other channels, you will protect your image of being bright and on top of things. Use your manager's time as efficiently and productively as your own.

If you feel that your manager does not give you *direction*, remember that your chief value lies in the extent of your ability to direct yourself. If you want to advance your career, you have to be able to take the initiative. Take this as an opportunity. You only need approval for your selected course of action.

If you are afraid to admit to mistakes, remember that errors are inevitable. Women especially have a problem believing this, and hesitate to jump in without preparation, afraid of making a mistake. Men, however, have more confidence to go through a time of error making to acquire their expertise. From an early age, women's efforts are focused on avoiding the errors that bring criticism. If this is the case, begin by acquiring as much experience as you can, and if you make an error, devise strategies to cover yourself. Learning from your errors is an important way of acquiring wisdom. Act quickly – do

---

5 Dickson A. *Women at Work: strategies for survival and success*. Kogan; 2000.

not procrastinate as mistakes are better tolerated when people see that you understand your error and that you have taken steps to correct it. If you have made the mistake of not dealing with a problem immediately, act as if the delay had never occurred.

You may be new to a job and feel it is not what you were *expecting*. If this is so, take care during the early days of your job, as job descriptions are often determined not in discussion during the interview, but in practice during the early days in the job. If you are asked to do anything that you do not consider is your remit, say so. Strong managers can bully their staff into something unacceptable. Establish your job description and then reject the new work, thus demonstrating that you are able to compromise and use your judgement, and that you will not be manipulated.

When you move into a new job, it is important for you to be seen as strong and confident. If you worry that you might be *failing*, take steps to recover your self-esteem. Appear in command: hand out short-term projects to your staff, so that you will quickly be able to judge their individual skills, and degree of competence and co-operativeness. Let everyone know that you are now in the judgement seat; that previous reputations do not count for very much. Be quick to praise and criticise. Do not show too much patience with those who do not deliver, as when you move in strongly, you are acting to minimise the possibilities of future trouble, and if people see you as a powerful force, they will think twice about engaging in office combat with you – and, instead, will seek out ways and means to ally themselves to you.

If you feel that you are not *achieving*, consider that one of the biggest single stumbling blocks to getting things done in any new job can be the inability to make the right contacts. Your first concern should be people: who will back your ideas or resist them, who is happy to see you come in and who resents you. Size up the different alliances before you get too friendly, and especially before you give work to staff. To win co-operation, court your colleagues assiduously, work on projects together, make lunch dates with them, throw them ideas that they can use in their own work, offer insights and ask for their advice.

MANAGING THE RELATIONSHIP WITH COLLEAGUES

This relationship depends on the task to be performed. You and your colleagues can be mutually interdependent, which means that neither could do the job alone. You may both work on the same projects simultaneously, so a continuous dialogue is needed; or you may be serially interdependent – one of you must finish a piece of the task before the other one can take it up; or you may work side by side with the same overall production objective.

Team working requires good problem-solving ability and a capacity to tolerate each other's working styles, be they quick, slow, meticulous or creative.

In this situation, you both keep checking your tolerances and expectations of each other. The skills required are those of collaboration and a sense of healthy, managed competition. You will need to be assertive – check how well you are interacting at intervals: 'How do you think we are working together?', 'I am satisfied with X, but feel we could improve on Y. How do you feel?' This strengthens equality, professional intimacy and mutual understanding, and communicates task-related thoughts and feelings. Socialisation meets important needs. For many people, it is a primary reason for enjoying work. Maximise your effectiveness and satisfaction by socialising 'up' as often as you can, socialising 'horizontally' frequently and, once, in a while socialise 'down', too.

The main issue in project working/serial interdependence is expectations. Be sure that you and your colleague agree on the quality specifications and your deadlines, and voice any concerns about the quality or timing of a colleague's work early: tell the other person what you appreciate about their work, reinstate your expectations and negotiate outcomes together.

MANAGING THE RELATIONSHIP WITH SUBORDINATES

There are particular dynamics of boss/subordinate relationships which you will need to be aware of. A boss is in a position of power, and sometimes a situation can develop where the manager's needs are largely met by his or her subordinates. If this occurs, he or she can feel good, free and satisfied in the relationship, but experience no need to share feelings, opinions and judgements. Implicitly, this keeps others doing all the other, 'difficult' feelings. In this situation, the subordinate spends a lot of energy assisting and supporting his or her boss, takes care of their perceived needs and may lose track of their own needs. They may become resentful, frustrated and angry, and begin to withhold their own feelings and thoughts because of perceived high risk.

A good boss should be aware of this power imbalance and work to know his or her subordinates well: their strengths and weaknesses; how they work under pressure and collaborate as team members; how they deal with ambiguity or unpredictability; their personality traits. Are they meticulous plodders? Sloppy but creative? Responsible, loyal, autonomous, ambitious?

If you do not know your staff, you cannot utilise their strengths and help to develop their potential. Get to know people: spend time with them, work and talk with them, observe and reflect. There are two critical components in the relationship with subordinates. First, a manager needs to communicate clearly with them; second, he or she must know how and when to delegate responsibility to them. Keep checking with the person on what they are hearing, on how they are feeling about the content of the communication. We know that the content is what is being said; the process is how it is being said.

DEVELOPING YOUR OWN MANAGEMENT SKILLS

Network

The grapevine reflects the opinions, hopes and anxieties of employees, and those who hope to know what is going on must learn to plug into it. Get out of your office, circulate and listen, identify the opinion leaders and gossips. Work to become trusted. To get information, you must give information. And it must be sound. Build friendships: you are a person, not just an employee or manager or someone out to get something.

Listen

As you go up in your career, listening to others becomes more and more crucial to your job. The executive must be a sensitive listener, not only for her or his own sake, but also because his or her position of authority affects other people's lives and careers. Be a good listener: establish an agreeable and pleasant atmosphere, so that the person you are listening to can feel relaxed. Be prepared to hear people through on their own terms: many of the messages that are worth listening to are not always presented well or in an inviting tone of voice. Even listen to those aspects that you disagree with. Make sure that you are well briefed on the subject to be discussed and avoid getting side-tracked, then listen for and summarise basic ideas – the only device for grasping what is being said and preventing misunderstandings.

Power and communication

People can communicate obliquely. In your organisation, learn the language and what it means. Power is often misunderstood.
➤ 'We're having an impromptu meeting. Come along if you want to.' If you are not at that meeting, you may miss something very important.
➤ 'Don't worry, but ...' means you should worry.
➤ If you are offered a challenge or an opportunity, you are going to be given a tough job.

Plan your career

Jobholders who succeed best map their careers; they do not leave everything to chance. Plan your career so that it fulfils your capacities, needs and dreams.
➤ What are your dreams? Where do you want to see yourself?
➤ What are your strengths and your assets, both in the job and out of it?
➤ What are your weaknesses? What kind of work do you fail in or wish to avoid? What areas do you need to strengthen yourself in? What areas of knowledge or self-cultivation must you pursue?
➤ What kind of lifestyle do you wish to achieve? What range of income and what kind of perks?

Do you have the skills to:
➤ plan strategically
➤ organise
➤ motivate, develop and give feedback
➤ clarify aims and objectives
➤ measure (formally and informally)
➤ self-assess
➤ analyse
➤ respond to and manage change
➤ delegate responsibility
➤ manage
  – resources
  – people
  – activities
  – information
  – energy
  – quality
  – projects?

For this, you will need knowledge: behavioural skills such as assertiveness, communication; influencing skills; complex cognitive abilities; self-knowledge; emotional resilience; and personal drive. Do you have the motivation to manage? Do you have a favourable attitude towards authority? Rebels never go far in any management hierarchy. Do you show a desire to compete – especially with peers? The desire to assert yourself and take charge? A desire to exert power and authority over people? A desire to behave in a distinctive and different way? Do you see taking visible and calculated risks as a challenge? A good manager is a good organiser, too, with a high tolerance for routines, repetitive, detailed paperwork, and an ability to pay attention to detail. These components are seen to be directly and reliably related to managerial success in terms of productivity, promotions, and pay.[6] Cultivate them if you wish to succeed.

KEY POINTS

➤ In the workplace, personal development refers to the methods and systems that support employee development and may include improving self-awareness, self-knowledge, and developing personal, professional strengths, talents and potential.

---

6 Miner J. *The Human Constraint: the coming shortage of managerial talent*. Bureau of National Affairs; 1994. p. 29. Fred Pryor Seminars. Pryor Resources, Inc. Available at: www.pryor.com (accessed April 2013).

➤ Personal development also includes developing other people through teaching, mentoring counselling, couching and supervising.

➤ To develop at work, you need to analyse the job you are aiming for, look at what the people at that level are doing and locate the key qualities and skills required. Pay good attention to yourself, your profession, your organisation.

➤ A good manager is seen to have valuable personal qualities – kindness, humour, respect, good listening skills – as well as excellent people skills – empathy, foresight, flexibility, generosity and tolerance – along with problem-solving ability and organisational and assertiveness skills.

➤ Weak managers are timid, weak or insecure. This shows in the ways that they undermine and invalidate, undercut self-confidence, and threaten or bully their staff. Poor managers are not accessible, do not achieve or provide direction, and are afraid to make mistakes.

➤ In the workplace, demonstrate key skills: the ability to think analytically, manage your time and prioritise your work. As well as being assertive and technologically numerate, show that you continually monitor and improve your own learning and performance.

➤ People succeed when they establish good relationships at work. Relationships, and good communication, are of the essence. Be strategic in developing important working relationships; understand your manager's and the organisation's responsibilities.

➤ Learn to qualify and quantify your productivity. Assess yourself and so increase your efficiency and effectiveness.

➤ Use management meetings to check that you are meeting objectives, understand required standards of performance and gain useful information about the needs of the organisation. Update your boss with information – gain feedback to improve your performance, confront difficult situations and solve problems, together.

➤ Team working requires good problem-solving ability, and a capacity to tolerate each other's working styles. The skills required are those of collaboration and a sense of healthy, managed competition.

➤ In developing our own management skills, we need to network, listen, be aware of the power bases and plan ahead. For this we need knowledge, motivation, tolerance and behavioural skills such as assertiveness, communication, influencing skills, complex cognitive abilities, self-knowledge, emotional resilience and personal drive.

FURTHER READING

Dickson A. *Women at Work: strategies for survival and success*. Kogan; 2000.

Guiliano M. *Women, Work, and the Art of Savoir Faire: business sense & sensibility*. Simon & Schuster Ltd; 2010.

Martin V, Henderson E. *Managing in Health and Social Care*. Routledge; 2001.

CHAPTER 13

Combatting stress

Stress is a pattern of physiological, behavioural, emotional and cognitive responses to real or imagined stimuli that are perceived as blocking a goal, or endangering, or otherwise threatening our well-being. The pressures in healthcare are growing relentlessly and remorselessly, and it is not uncommon for public sector workers to feel some of these emotional and cognitive responses. It is reassuring to know that the Health and Safety Executive has made certain that our employers have a responsibility to us in managing both our physical and mental health at work, and to achieve this has put in place a raft of preventative and support strategies to help deal with the unprecedented rise in stress-related illness in the workforce.

External stressors have different effects on different people. Clearly, those working in front line services, such as accident and emergency, rapid response, cancer services, ambulance drivers, or anyone dealing with potential trauma on a daily basis (terminal illnesses, baby deaths, breaking bad news) will have unqualifiable daily stressors to deal with. These stresses are intrinsic to the job. However, many people manage to work with such personal trauma on a daily basis for many years, cheerfully, capably and competently. Many others are ill-equipped for dealing with the minor stressors, hassles and irritations that life throws at us.

So stress is a personal perception and response, the resilience to which is based on personality and skills, which can be learned and developed. This chapter will assist you in recognising the signs and symptoms of stress, and give you some strategies for dealing with it. We look at what stress is, some of the common causes and how it can be important. It includes some practical guidelines for managing stress – how you can help yourself and involve other people to assist you. The symptoms of stress are reversible. If you are experiencing stress, it will be important for your immediate and long-term health and well-being not to ignore the signs, but to work assertively to alleviate or combat the stressful feelings.

Anyone working in healthcare understands work-a-day stress responses. If asked, the majority of healthcare workers report that administration, dealing with workload and the pressure from unhappy people chasing reports/results/cancelled appointments are the strongest predictors of them feeling stressed or depressed. Many work more than their contracted hours per week, not always paid. The stresses vary for each discipline. Front line services have their own methods for managing their particular stresses, with supervision and debriefing forming a cornerstone to stress management. Common stress-inducing activities for office workers in general practice are finding locums and future planning; for clinicians, it may be the pressure to fit in a certain number of patient contacts per day, plus the associated pressure to respond promptly from partner agencies. These stresses – work overload – are not intrinsic to the role, but due in part to the organisational role being played. The two most cited contemporary models for occupational stress are an imbalance between effort and reward, and work which combines the extremes of high demand and low control.[1]

Current estimates are that up to 30% of all GP consultations are stress related.[2] Unpublished medical opinion considers this to be a conservative estimate, and cites that possibly up to 80% of all diseases have psychosomatic origins. Other estimates within healthcare show high levels of burnout among inner-city GPs in particular,[3] with 44% feeling drained and exhausted and 42% depersonalising patients. Younger GPs seem particularly vulnerable. The statistics speak for themselves: a 2004 survey conducted by the American Psychological Association found that:

➤ 45% of workers report that job insecurity has a significant impact on stress levels
➤ 61% of workers list heavy workloads as a significant impact on stress levels
➤ 25% of workers have taken a day off to cope with stress
➤ 54% of workers are concerned about health problems due to stress.[4]

Of course, many people do not seek professional help for their stress-related difficulties. However, of those that do, of note are the recent psychological services (Improving Access to Psychological Therapies, IAPT) targets for 2010/11, which include 900,000 people treated for common mental health problems, with 50% of them 'moving towards recovery'. Overall, the aim is to establish an IAPT site in every primary care trust in the UK by 2011, providing access to psychological treatment for at least half of the UK population.

---

1 Vincenti G, consultant psychiatrist. In: Teachers and stress. *The Times*. 2012 May 15. p. 23.
2 www.scotland.gov.uk/Publications/2006/11/30164829/5 (accessed April 2013).
3 Bhattacharya S. GP burnout poses threat to implementation of NHS Plan. *Pulse*. 2001 Jul. p. 3.
4 www.ourstressfullives.com/stress-statistics.html (accessed April 2013).

SIGNS AND SYMPTOMS OF STRESS

EXERCISE 1

Consider whether you:
➤ feel guilty when relaxing
➤ feel irritable, impatient, frustrated
➤ have difficulty concentrating, worry continually
➤ feel endlessly tired or suffer from niggling physical complaints
➤ feel disorientated when the day's work finishes
➤ feel increasingly cynical and disenchanted with your work
➤ feel emotionally exhausted and increasingly forgetful
➤ are working harder and harder and accomplishing less and less
➤ depersonalise: treat patients as impersonal objects
➤ feel you are not achieving as well as you were
➤ feel continually tense
➤ are smoking or drinking more than usual
➤ experience a dry mouth, sweaty palms or an upset stomach in difficult situations
➤ experience work as a series of crises that you never seem to solve
➤ have difficulty getting to sleep or wake early; lie awake thinking, yet be unable to reach decisions.

You will not be alone: a 2009 survey conducted by the American Psychological Association[5] found that many adults reported feeling the following physical effects of stress:

47% reported lying awake at night
45% reported irritability or anger
43% reported fatigue
40% reported lack of interest, motivation or energy
34% reported headaches
34% reported feeling sad or depressed
32% reported feeling as though they could cry
27% reported upset stomach or indigestion.

Stress could be described as a concept about a condition that evokes these feelings of strain, pressure, anxiety, overwhelmed, overall irritability, insecurity, nervousness, social withdrawal, loss of appetite, depression, poor decision making or panic attacks. Chronic stress and a lack of coping resources can often lead to the development of psychological issues such as depression and anxi-

---

5 Ibid.

ety.[6] This is particularly true of daily stressors, which tend to have a more negative impact on health because they occur daily over long periods, thus evoking a daily physiological response, which takes its toll on our bodies, depleting energy.

Physiologically, it is not uncommon to demonstrate symptoms of exhaustion, high or low blood pressure, skin problems, insomnia, lack of sexual desire or sexual dysfunction, migraine, gastrointestinal problems leading to constipation or diarrhoea, and, for women, menstrual problems. It may cause more serious conditions such as lowered immunity and heart problems. How often do you experience these symptoms, and how often do you talk about them? If often, you may be suffering from some of the physical and emotional effects of stress.

There is no doubt that we could be happier, healthier and more productive if stress free. Medical problems are not inevitable, and there are many techniques to assist. Most of us will feel that some of the statements above apply some of the time. Indeed, stress needs to be part of everyday life as it helps keep us alert and out of danger. In small doses, it can create a 'high' where challenges are enjoyed, and it accounts for feelings of excitement and optimism when a new venture is started. Thus everyday pressures, or small amounts of stress, may be desired, beneficial, and even healthy and productive. Positive stress helps to improve athletic performance. It is also a factor in motivation, adaptation and reaction to the environment; but clearly, excessive amounts of stress may lead to many problems in the body that could be harmful.

Stress could be something external and related to the environment,[7] such as the reality of an increased workload, but may not be directly created by external events. If situations remind a person of prior threatening events, stressful feelings can be evoked. Here it is the internal perceptions that cause an individual to have anxiety/negative emotions surrounding a situation. Humans experience stress, or perceive things as threatening, when they do not believe that their resources for coping with obstacles (stimuli, people, situations, etc.) are enough for what the circumstances demand. When we think the demands being placed on us exceed our ability to cope, we then perceive stress. What we then need to do is to learn how to develop resilience and capability.

Any new life event or change does create stress, but we often feel the positive rather than the negative changes. We experience the same physical and mental alertness when we are about to embark on a physically demanding venture such as preparing for a sporting event, and it is clear that in these circumstances a degree of stress is essential.

---

6 Kemeny ME. The psychobiology of stress. *Current Directions in Psychological Science*. 2003; **12**(4): 124–9.

7 Jones F, Bright J, Clow A. *Stress: myth, theory and research*. Pearson Education; 2001. p. 4.

PHYSIOLOGICAL REACTIONS TO STRESS

In a potentially dangerous or threatening situation, our bodies automatically react: senses sharpen; adrenaline floods into our bloodstream; we prepare for action. Instincts have primed us for self-survival, in a classic stress response. However, this bodily preparation is often unnecessary. Our bodies are primed to expect physical attack, and the physical responses experienced are a legacy from a time when we had to fight for our lives. It takes a good while for the body to return to a calm equilibrium. Our bodies cannot tell the difference between events that are actual threats to survival and events that are present in thoughts alone. As our society has developed, we have invented situations that are impossible to deal with physically. We cannot escape from a traffic jam; we cannot satisfactorily verbally abuse a computer when it makes an error. We are simply stuck with the feelings and the exaggerated bodily reactions.

Stress, whether acute or chronic, releases an array of hormones that provide quick energy. Two of these, adrenalin and cortisol, are potent inhibitors of the immune system. Other changes occur. The heart rate increases, with a concomitant increase in blood pressure. Our internal organs cease to work effectively as blood flow to them is reduced. The chemical build up in our muscles does not dissipate easily: small nodules appear, classically around the neck and shoulder area. The frequent surges in blood pressure can lead to heart disease; stomach tensions to ulcers. The hormonal residue can cause irritation, frustration, impatience and mood swings. We then overeat to soothe ourselves, take drugs to ease the upset stomach, use tobacco, drugs or alcohol artificially to calm or deaden the experience.

In terms of measuring the body's response to stress, psychologists tend to use Han Selye's general adaption syndrome.[8] This model is also often referred to as the classic stress response. It revolves around the concept of homeostasis, where in response to stressors, the body seeks to return to its equilibrium state, or the normal level of stress resistance. During the alarm phase, the body begins to build up resistance to the stressor beyond normal resistance levels and mobilises the sympathetic nervous system to meet the immediate threat: the body reacts by releasing adrenal hormones that produce a boost in energy, tense muscles, reduced sensitivity to pain, the shutting down of digestion and a rise in blood pressure. In the resistance phase, the body attempts to resist or cope with a persistent stressor that cannot be avoided. The physiological responses of the alarm phase continue and make the body much more vulnerable to other stressors.[9] The body continues building up resistance throughout the stage of resistance, until either its resources are depleted, leading to the exhaustion phase, or the stressful stimulus is removed. This three-phase

---

8   Selye H. Stress without distress. *Ann Intern Med.* 1974; 81(5): 716.
9   Gottlieb B. *Coping with Chronic Stress*. Plenum Press; 1997.

response is designed to help humans in life or death situations, but all types of stressors can trigger this response. A stress response results in elevated physiological arousal, often associated with the release of stress hormones such as cortisol.

This physiological stress response involves high levels of sympathetic nervous system arousal, often referred to as the 'fight or flight' response, it is this that causes the release of endorphins, increased heart and respiration rates, cessation of digestive processes, secretion of adrenaline, arteriole dilation and constriction of veins. This high level of arousal is unnecessary for coping adequately with micro-stressors, yet it is the response pattern seen in humans, which often leads to health issues commonly associated with high levels of stress.[10]

The physiological response to stress demands much of the body's energy and resources, and has great impact on disease and risk for disease. When the body's energy is used to respond to minor (or major) stressors, the immune system's ability to function properly is compromised.[11] This makes the individual more susceptible to physical illnesses such as a cold or flu. Stressful events also often result in insomnia, impaired sleeping and health complaints.[12]

THE CAUSES OF STRESS

Types of stressors

In 1988, Cohen, *et al.* examined some of the more common experiences defined by people as stressors, and identified that any physical or psychological event, experience or environmental stimuli, if perceived as a threat or challenge to the individual, may be a stressor.[13] We have seen that these stressors can make individuals more prone to both physical and psychological problems. Stressors are more likely to affect an individual's health when they are chronic, highly disruptive or perceived as uncontrollable.

Cohen's team classified the different types of stressors into three categories:
➤ crises/catastrophes
➤ major life events
➤ daily hassles/micro-stressors.

---

10 Ogden J. *Health Psychology: a textbook*. 4th ed. McGraw-Hill; 2007.

11 Greubel J, Kecklund G. *The Impact of Organizational Changes on Work Stress, Sleep, Recovery and Health*. Industrial Health. Department for Psychology, University of Fribourg; 2009.

12 Schlotz W, Yim I, Zoccola P, *et al.* The perceived stress reactivity scale: measurement invariance, stability, and validity in three countries. *Psychol Assess*. 2011; **23**(1): 80–94.

13 Cohen S, Frank E, Doyle WJ, *et al.* Types of stressors that increase susceptibility to the common cold in healthy adults. *Health Psychology*. 1998; **17**(3): 211–13.

Crises/catastrophes are the unforeseen and unpredictable events, such as natural disasters, that are completely out of the control of the individual. Though rare in occurrence, this type of stressor naturally and typically causes a great deal of stress in a person's life. Common examples of *major life events* include the death of a loved one and the birth of a child, events that can be either positive or negative. Positive events generally, as one would expect, do not cause stress, but the length of time since occurrence is a factor in whether stress occurs and how much stress it causes. Events that have occurred within the past month generally are not linked to stress or illness, while chronic events that occurred more than several months ago are linked to stress and illness.

The *daily hassles/micro-stressors* category includes the most commonly occurring types of stressor in an individual's everyday life, and the ones we are most interested in here, including daily annoyances and minor hassles such as decision making, meeting deadlines, traffic jams, encounters with those we find difficult or are in conflict with. Daily stressors, however, are different for each individual, as not everyone perceives a certain event as stressful. For example, most people find public speaking to be stressful, but a seasoned speaker most likely will not. Within this, decision making itself can cause stress, whether the person is choosing between two equally attractive options (approach-approach conflict), two equally unattractive options (avoidance-avoidance conflict), or where a person is forced to choose whether or not to partake in something that has both attractive and unattractive traits, such as whether to attend university or take a gap year (where decisions around loans/employment/friendships make this an approach/avoidance conflict).

Stress scales

Stress scales are lists of life events that can contribute to illness in an individual. The most frequently used is the Social Readjustment Rating Scale, or SRRS.[14] Originally developed by psychiatrists 1967, the scale lists 43 events that can cause stress.

To calculate one's score, add up the number of 'life change units' for events that have occurred in the past year. A score of more than 300 means that individual is at risk for illness; a score between 150 and 299 means the risk of illness is moderate; and a score under 150 means that there is only a slight risk of illness.[15]

14 Carlson NR, Heth CD. *Psychology: the science of behaviour*. 4th Canadian ed. with MyPsychLab. Pearson Education Canada; 2010. p. 526.

15 Cohen, Frank, Doyle, *et al.*, note 13 above. Carlson, Heth, note 14 above.

Life event	Life change units
Death of a spouse	100
Divorce	73
Marital separation	65
Imprisonment	63
Death of a close family member	63
Personal injury or illness	53
Marriage	50
Dismissal from work	47
Marital reconciliation	45
Retirement	45
Change in health of a family member	44
Pregnancy	40
Sexual difficulties	39
Gain a new family member	39
Business readjustment	39
Change in financial state	38
Death of a close friend	37
Change to different line of work	36
Change in frequency of arguments	35
Major debt/mortgage arrears	32
Foreclosure of mortgage or loan	30
Change in responsibilities at work	29
Child leaving home	29
Trouble with in-laws	29
Outstanding personal achievement	28
Spouse starts or stops work	26
Begin or end school	26
Change in living conditions	25
Revision of personal habits	24
Trouble with boss	23
Change in working hours or conditions	20
Change in residence	20
Change in schools	20
Change in recreation	19
Change in church activities	19
Change in social activities	18
Minor mortgage or loan	17

Life event	Life change units
Change in sleeping habits	16
Change in number of family reunions	15
Change in eating habits	15
Vacation	13
Christmas	12
Minor violation of law	11

So stress, as a definition, is often used incorrectly. Stressors are events, situations, stimuli, etc. that can cause people to perceive threat, leading them to experience anxiety, feeling overwhelmed or other negative emotions. Thus, as we have seen, it is not these events, these traumas, conversations, etc., that cause the stress, but instead our perception of how we will be able to cope with these stimuli.

Physiologically, day-to-day/chronic stressors have a greater negative impact on individuals' health than do more acute, traumatic stressors, which generally have a start and an end point (*see* classic stress response, above). For example, daily stressors such as dealing with traffic, completing assignments, etc., cause more harm to one's health in the long run than do stressors such as a death in the family, marriage, etc.

IDENTIFYING STRESSORS

EXERCISE 2

List your own causes: begin to develop self-awareness.

Write down your personal stress triggers

EXERCISE 3

Identifying personal stressors. How vulnerable are you to stress?[16]

Score each item: 1 = almost always   5 = never.

	Score
I eat at least one balanced meal a day.	1
I get seven to eight hours' sleep at least four nights a week.	1
I give and receive affection regularly.	1
I have at least one relative within 50 miles on whom I can rely.	1
I exercise to the point of perspiration at least twice a week.	5
I smoke less than 10 cigarettes a day.	1
I take fewer than five alcoholic drinks a week.	1
I am the appropriate weight for my height.	5
I have an income adequate to meet basic expenses.	1
I get strength from my religious beliefs.	4
I regularly attend club or social activities.	3
I have a network of friends to confide in about personal matters.	1
I am in good health.	1
I am able to speak openly about my feelings when angry or worried.	1
I have regular conversations with the people I live with about domestic problems, for example, chores, money and daily living worries.	1
I do something for fun at least once a week.	1
I am able to organise my time effectively.	2
I drink fewer than three cups of coffee (tea, cola) a day.	1
I take quiet time for myself during the day.	1
Total	33

To get your score, add up your figures and subtract 20. Any number over 30 indicates a vulnerability to stress. You are seriously vulnerable if you score

---

16 Test developed by psychologists Lyn Miller and Alma Dell Smith from Boston University Medical Centre, 1984.

between 50 and 75, and extremely vulnerable if your score is over 75. Time to review your lifestyle?

EXERCISE 4

Our workplace environment and conditions can contribute to stress. Mark off which of these factors are contributing to your stress.[17]

Workplace environment

➤ Poor light levels and air quality.
➤ Unmanaged interruptions.
➤ Infrequent breaks.
➤ Lack of privacy.
➤ Low resources.
➤ Staff shortfalls.
➤ Essential travel.

The work

➤ Does everyone understand the nature of your work?
➤ Work overload or underload?
➤ Are you adequately trained for the job?
➤ Are there any specific demands made of you that are unusual?
➤ Are your work boundaries defined or vague?
➤ Is there enough variety in your work?
➤ Is your work developing?

Relationships

➤ Are you well managed?
➤ Do you have good relationships with your colleagues?

Rewards

➤ Are you paid adequately for the job?
➤ Are you appraised?
➤ Is your work acknowledged?

Organisational culture

➤ What are the expected behaviours of your organisation and do you fit in?
➤ What is the extent of communication and consultation?
➤ Are there any internal power struggles?
➤ Office politics?
➤ Conflicts with values?

---

17 Collins G. *Spotlight on Stress*. Vision House; 1985.

➤ Is change imposed or managed?
➤ Are there frequent structural changes?
➤ Are new technologies and skills being introduced?

Career development

➤ Promotion prospects?
➤ Redundancy?
➤ Retirement looming?
➤ Training opportunities?

Some of the most common forms of *stress* at work have been identified.[18]

➤ Intrinsic to the job – working conditions.
➤ Role in the organisation – underload or overload.
➤ Relationships at work – especially with management.
➤ Career development – especially in mid-life.
➤ Organisational structure and climate – rules and regulations.
➤ Home/work interface – especially the growth of duel career families.

Stress is exacerbated when we have a taste of power but cannot wield much influence. Having severe financial or partnership problems creates additional mental and emotional strains; relationships become fraught and easily break down, which creates a new cycle of problems. Public sector workers have the additional strain of anticipating unwelcome or unknown change in their job environment with every new change of government. Managers and practitioners have different stresses, but both experience lack of time and work overload, have to balance loyalties and are sandwiched between demands from the government, commissioners, doctors, staff and clients. This is an uncomfortable position. We fear voicing our disquiet. There is the risk of voicing dissatisfaction to superiors, as workers want to appear in control. If ambitious, there is a perceived need to keep the status quo, to not appear weak. However, unless this is tackled assertively, it can create its own tensions: the avoidance/avoidance conflict mentioned above. This can lead to feelings of fighting a silent battle, which can push the individual further and further into a corner of their own making.

Undoubtedly, public sector workers also face an unprecedented amount of change throughout their working lives. While organisational change undoubtedly brings with it the possibility of creativity in the form of developing new ideas and innovative services, it is also likely to heighten anxiety in the face

---

18 Cooper C, Cooper R, Eaker L. *Living with Stress*. Penguin; 1988.

of risk, uncertainty and loss of familiar ways of working. The requirements for service redesign and redeployment, as well as managing ever-increasing numbers of patients, all serve to heighten anxiety within healthcare teams about their capacity adequately to meet public and governmental expectations.

At a clinical level, too, there are anxieties about the capacity of some staff groups' capacity to carry out and sustain clinical work with psychologically distressed individuals. A recent qualitative research study within psychological services showed how some low-intensity workers were struggling to cope with patients becoming tearful, angry or demanding, and how they found the emotional impact of clinical work unexpectedly challenging and draining.[19] Some researchers have suggested that in uncertain or complex environments, where anxiety levels are high, the mental state of the group may become driven by the need for emotional security.[20] We sometimes see this in group and team dynamics, where groups working under intense strain or psychological pressure set up a 'them and us' mentality, resulting in group dependencies, pairings and cliques. Thus primary care is angry with secondary care, the NHS believes that its local authority colleagues could be doing a better job, and social workers feel that the Child and Adolescent Mental Health Service (CAMHS) never accepts referrals, etc. Each team develops such defences against the anxiety of uncertainty, chaos and 'not knowing'.

Such primitive anxieties sometimes lead organisations to construct particular routines and procedures that ultimately sabotage the very tasks they are required to carry out. Group practices, and individual burn out, lead people to become increasingly reluctant to care for patients. A very early (1959) study found that nurses experienced enormous emotional difficulties in working with and handling sick, dying and injured patients.[21] The study identified a number of working practices, such as strict routines and division of workload; the idealisation of the professional, 'detached' nurse untouched by the death of a patient; the identification of patients by number rather than by name; the reduction in responsibility via delegation to superiors; and the avoidance of change.

These practices, while serving to reduce anxiety at both an organisational and personal level, then, paradoxically reduced the nurses' emotional investment and satisfaction in relationships with their patients. Inhibition of

---

19 Rizq R, Hewey M, Salvo L, *et al.* Reflective voices: primary care mental health workers' experiences in training and practice. *Primary Healthcare Research and Development*. 2010; **11**: 72–86.

20 Bion W. *Experiences in Groups and Other Papers*. Tavistock; 1961. Bollas C. *Being a Character: psychoanalysis and self experience*. Routledge; 1992.

21 Menzies Lyth I. Social systems as a defence against anxiety. *Human Relations*. 1959; **13**: 95–121. In: Rizq R. IATP, anxiety and envy: a psychoanalytic view of NHS primary care mental health services today. *British Journal of Psychotherapy*. 2011; **27**(1): 37–55.

the nurses' capacities and creative energies led to high levels of doubt and job dissatisfaction, which in turn led to a rapid and destabilising staff turnover at the hospital. This then further undermined the development of close and effective working relationships, which could have gone some way to offset the level of anxiety within the institution.

When risk-assessing to see how stressed we are, another way of analysing our propensity to stress is to look at four variables:

➤ the demands on our life
➤ our relationships
➤ the level of control we have
➤ our support systems.

The demands may be reports, targets, expectations – at home these will be different. Our relationships may be positive or negative, and include relationships with colleagues, parents, carers, our role models at work. We need to feel autonomous, that we are in control. We need to develop our support structures: peers, friends, managers, supervisors, our team.

It is important that our work role is valued, that we are appreciated and told so. It is also important that we have the skills and knowledge to perform our job, and that we are clear about our job description and the boundaries of our role. With job reduction common, we may be conflicted within that role, as we may be both manager and colleague, a clinical manager, a professional and line manager. These are issues we need to be aware of, and, if necessary, seek help on.

PERSONALITIES AND STRESS

Studies have shown that perceived chronic stress and the hostility associated with more aggressive, driven personalities are often associated with much higher risks of cardiovascular disease, occurring because of the compromised immune system as well as the high levels of arousal in the sympathetic nervous system.[22] This more driven personality 'type' used to be termed 'Type A' personality,[23] and its counterpart, the more passive, relaxed, easy-going 'Type B' personality. However, these terms are now formally discredited in the literature: type theories in general have been criticised as overly simplistic and incapable of assessing the degrees of difference in human personality. Despite this, the terms are in the public consciousness and so are still in common use. They

---

22 Pastorino E, Doyle-Portillo S. *What is Psychology?* 2nd ed. Thompson Higher Education; 2009.
23 Friedman M, Rosenman R. Association of specific overt behaviour pattern with blood and cardiovascular findings. *Journal of the American Medical Association.* 1959; **169**: 1286–96.

are used here to describe groups of behaviours that readers may recognise in themselves.

Psychologists today have broadened their interest beyond this behaviour analysis, and current research is focused on resilience: the study of the factors that allow individuals to cope with stress and evade most health and illness problems associated with high levels of stress. There is the understanding that, despite intrinsic and extrinsic stressors, it is possible for individuals to exhibit hardiness – a term referring to the ability to be both chronically stressed and healthy.[24] This may be true of front-line workers (accident and emergency workers, police, paramedics, fire-fighters) who face significant trauma on a daily basis. Another aspect being investigated is that of positive psychology.[25] Authentic happiness is a branch of psychology that focuses on the empirical study of such things as positive emotions, strengths-based character and healthy institutions. Thus there is a recognition that certain personality types have a higher resilience to stress.

High achievers

EXAMPLE A

> 'There must be something on my list that I can work on immediately, I suppose that I am a "Type A" personality; the sort you might call a high achiever. I enjoy a challenge and am industrious.'

This individual is tackling her problems constructively – she has listed her personal stressors. This part of her list focuses on work:

1 time wasters
2 the phone
3 having projects interfered with
4 partner B
5 overrunning meetings
6 constant interruptions
7 ? the future and uncertainty if I change my job.

This worker has identified that there are some things that she likes doing which cause her some degree of stress. This is to be expected – life and living are stressful. One of the ways that she could reduce her stress levels is by managing her time more effectively. The other is to look at those areas of her life that cannot

---

24 Kobasa SC. The hardy personality: toward a social psychology of stress and health. In: Sanders GS, Suls J, editors. *Social Psychology of Health and Illness*. Lawrence Erlbaum Assoc.; 1982. pp. 1–25.
25 Seligman M. *Authentic Happiness*. Positive Psychology Center, University of Pennsylvania. Available at: www.authentichappiness.org (accessed April 2013).

be so easily changed, and change her attitudes towards them. Once the list is broken down into manageable portions, it is easier to identify a problem and put things into perspective.

➤ What can you can give up?
➤ What you can change easily?
➤ What do you need help with?

If you are hard-driving, aggressive or assertive, you will have your own problems: you are sometimes ruthless, but more often than not you are praised and rewarded for your activities. You may:

➤ be an opportunist
➤ push yourself to the limit
➤ treat tasks unnecessarily as emergencies
➤ feel guilty when relaxing
➤ be easily bored
➤ be competitive
➤ be high-achieving
➤ be impatient and ambitious for success
➤ always seek approval from others
➤ believe that success comes from doing things at the fastest possible rate.

Friedman described Type A individuals as ambitious, rigidly organised, sometimes hostile, status conscious, impatient, irritable, short-fused, easily exasperated, competitive, achievement-driven and obsessed with time management.[26] People with this trait are often high-achieving workaholics who multi-task, push themselves with deadlines, and hate both delays and ambivalence: traits you may see in yourself, among others. However, as Pastorino and Doyle-Portillo found,[27] Type A behaviour is not a good predictor of coronary heart disease; it is the hostility which is the significant risk factor. Thus, it is a high level of expressed anger and hostility, not the other elements of Type A behaviour, that constitute the problem.

Those that tend to work in fast-moving jobs which require an extrovert personality and also quick decision-making may chose to manage in an environment of rapid change and development. In this, the personality attributes can be destructive. In the struggle to achieve more in less time, it is often at the expense of others, and even your own health. Informal observation shows that behavioural characteristics may include: walking and eating rapidly; trying to do two or more things at the same time; not allowing for unforeseen

26 Friedman M. *Type A Behavior: its diagnosis and treatment*. Plenum Press (Kluwer Academic Press); 1996. p. 31ff.
27 Pastorino, Doyle-Portillo, note 22 above.

events; trying to hurry people's speech/finishing their sentences; treating people as rivals/competitors rather than friends or colleagues; and being subject to nervous tics or gestures (e.g. incessantly running fingers through the hair). These behaviour traits are not always easy to be around and, for this alone, it is worth considering managing these aspects more constructively, through counselling, therapy, mediation or Mindfulness[28] techniques, for example. Identifying the areas that feel uncontrollable is a good start. Although there are some things that we cannot control – like the future, which can not be altered – attitudes can, and it is this area that we shall examine next. We need to believe in our own power, and believe that we can get our future exactly how we want it.

Moderate personality types

If you identify with the Type B personality – a less extreme, quieter, more passive type – consider these beliefs, cited by Dickson,[29] that you may hold about yourself. Then question their validity, and reframe them constructively.

> ➤ I must be loved or liked by everyone, people should love me.
> ➤ I must be perfect in all I do.
> ➤ All the people with whom I work or live must be perfect.
> ➤ I have little control over what happens to me.
> ➤ It is easier to avoid facing difficulties than to deal with them.
> ➤ Disagreement and conflict are a disaster and must be avoided at all costs.
> ➤ People, including me, do not change.
> ➤ Some people are always good, others bad.
> ➤ The world should be perfect and it is terrible that it is not.
> ➤ People are fragile and need to be protected from the truth.
> ➤ Other people exist to make us happy and we cannot be happy unless they do so.
> ➤ Crises are invariably and entirely destructive and no good can come of them.
> ➤ Somewhere is the perfect job, the perfect solution and perfect partner, and all we need to do is search for them.
> ➤ We should not have problems. If we do, it indicates we are incompetent.
> ➤ There is only one way – the true way.

---

28 Kabat-Zinn J. *Full Catastrophe Living: how to cope with stress, pain and illness using Mindfulness meditation.* Piatkus; 2001. Alidina S. *Mindfulness for Dummies.* John Wiley & Sons; 2010.

29 Dickson A. *A Woman in Your Own Right: assertiveness and you.* Revised 30th anniversary ed. Quartet Books; 2012.

Challenge this destructive self-talk through cognitive reframing techniques. A cognitive behaviour therapy (CBT) approach focuses our thinking and behaviour in order to help us overcome any emotional and behavioural problems. Remember the last time you felt bad about something: angry, jealous, resentful, etc. What were you telling yourself? We often have a series of very destructive beliefs, many of which have been handed down from our parents. They are destructive because they mean that we set impossibly high targets for ourselves that are impossible to attain. Think about some of these beliefs, and then challenge them logically. Destructive talk is judgemental, and may well include unfair condemnation of yourself.

> Destructive: 'I must be liked or loved by everyone.'
>
> Constructive: 'I don't like everyone, so why should everyone like me? I love and am loved by a chosen few.'

> Destructive: 'Disagreement and conflict are a disaster and must be avoided at all costs.'
>
> Constructive: 'I can learn from conflicts. It is possible to disagree and still remain friends.'

> Destructive: 'I must be perfect.'
>
> Constructive: 'Perfection is impossible to attain. The world is not perfect, nor can we be.'

> Destructive: 'Other people exist to make us happy and we cannot be happy unless they do.'
>
> Constructive: 'Happiness comes from within.'

Friedman describes Type B individuals in perfect contrast to those with Type A personalities.[30] People with Type B personalities are generally apathetic, patient, relaxed, easy-going, but also have no sense of time schedule, have poor organisation skills, and at times lack an overriding sense of urgency. If these traits are linked with suppressing emotional expression, and denying strong emotional reactions, it will be less easy for the individual to cope successfully with stress. There maybe a tendency to react by giving up, linked with feelings of hopelessness and helplessness. It has been commonly thought that this type of response may lead to a suppression of our immune systems, leading to

---

30 Friedman, note 26 above.

more significant disease,[31] but again much of this early research has since been discredited, and much more research is needed. However, attitude to health and well-being does seem to be important, and so more moderate or passive personalities may benefit from:

➤ talking more about feelings
➤ writing in a personal journal about the hardest emotions
➤ sharing a stress interview with a colleague
➤ identifying and extending support networks
➤ learning and applying some counselling skills
➤ challenging destructive self-talk (cognitive reframing).

Neurological diversity

People vary a lot in their ability to hold on to information, update awareness, and seek stimulation, novelty and excitement. If you are aware that you are someone who constantly updates their working memory, you may have a hard time screening out irrelevant and distracting stimuli. If your attention seeking is high, you may be likely to over-focus or obsess, and easily get into sensory overload. If this is you, try to develop good concentration skills, the ability to divide your attention and focus on what is really important in a situation. This way you will gain the mental flexibility needed to assimilate and accommodate new situations.

STRESS MANAGEMENT

The NHS is developing many excellent treatment options to reduce the impact of stress and support people through using a stepped care approach such as that being developed in Scotland,[32] or providing a range of appropriate treatment options by making counselling and CBT more available through the wider availability of psychological services (IAPT services). We are living through a time of unprecedented change in the field of psychological therapies. The Labour government's response to the 2004 Layard report, *Mental Health: Britain's biggest social problem*,[33] was to fund and implement the Improving Access to Psychological Therapies (IAPT) programme. This incorporates the stepped care model proposed within the National Institute for Health and Care Excellence (NICE) guidelines, and advocates the introduction of large numbers of mental health practitioners in the NHS delivering 'low-intensity' guided

---

31 Temoshok L. Personality, coping style, emotion, and cancer. Towards an integrative model. *Cancer Surveys*. 1987; 6: 545–67.
32 National Evaluation Report published in 2006. Available at: www.scotland.gov.uk/Publications/2006/11/30164829/5 (accessed April 2013).
33 Layard R. *Mental Health: Britain's biggest social problem*. Department of Health; 2004.

self-help interventions, computerised CBT, and signposting to voluntary sector services alongside 'high intensity' therapeutic work, with the 'talking' or CBTs.

What follows are some of the approaches used by therapists and work and well-being practitioners: developing resilience, therapeutic techniques, problem-solving skills, and behavioural and lifestyle changes.

Developing resilience

As we have discussed, resilience is based part on personality, part on skills. For an assessment of your own resilience levels based on personality, try the online tools developed by www.robertsoncooper.com/iresilience This company, which advises workplaces and individuals on stress management techniques, notes that once we reach adulthood, our personalities remain relatively stable, but that our levels of resilience can vary considerably. Fortunately, everyone has the ability to build and maintain their levels of resilience. The *i-resilience* report reveals which of the four key components users naturally draw on for resilience – confidence, adaptability, purposefulness and the need for social support. It provides an understanding of personal resilience and gives examples of how this could impact on users' responses to demanding work situations. It is possible to build on existing areas of strength, and to develop resilience, and this is the line that the employers are encouraging us to go down, given that stress can be avoided entirely, both at home and at work. We have to build the skills required to deal with it.

Resilience helps us to cope with adversity, rebalance, adapt to change and the uncertainty of life. We can help to build resilience in ourselves and our organisations by building morale, encouraging each other and supporting well-being. If we identify with our professional roles, have ownership of any changes, and have an open and transparent management structure, this helps to build our workplace coping skills: these factors affect absenteeism, productivity, cost effectiveness and customer satisfaction.

The four main factors that help to build individual resilience are as follows.
1　**Confidence:** being positive, assertive, self-aware, emotionally intelligent.
2　**Social support:** the varied feedback from friends and colleagues which lends itself to increasing our perspective and reduces isolation.
3　**Purposefulness:** motivation, determination and drive.
4　**Adaptability:** the ability to problem solve, to rise to challenges, to adapt to, and enjoy, change.

What helps is the ability to maintain a sense of humour, flexibility, optimism and see challenges as opportunities. We need clear direction, drive and persistence. We need the confidence to manage our own self-esteem and emotions. These positive traits help to keep us 'topped up' and help to guard us against emotionally draining, or taxing, situations. They help us to flourish.

Involving others

The following series of exercises[34] describe some simple techniques that may help to improve emotional resilience.

EXERCISE 5

➤ Talk about your feelings with someone close to you.
➤ Share your problems with the people who are important to you, without overburdening either yourself or them. A problem shared is a problem halved.

One, more formal method is to write in and exchange personal journals, in which you identify and describe your feelings and attitudes in more detail. You and your chosen partner/friend spend five or 10 minutes a day writing down some of the emotions and feelings generated by difficult situations. Then spend another 10 minutes exchanging your thoughts. It is often easier to expose yourself on paper – and the paper does not interrupt, look critical or bored. It may be easier to decide on a series of topics to write about, such as the following.

What is the nicest thing that has ever happened to you?
What is the most devastating?
How do you feel about growing old?
What is the hardest emotion to share?
Do the words 'commitment' and 'responsibility' scare you, and if not, why not?
Who does/has provided you with the most emotional support in your lifetime?
What is the hardest emotion for you to share?

EXERCISE 6

Choose an adjective to discuss what each of these words mean to you. Try to recall the incidents when these emotions have surfaced.

Friendship Hurt Inadequate Domineering Confident
Uncertain Unappreciated Sympathy Proud

---

34 Powell J. *The Secret of Staying in Love*. Resources for Christian Living; 1996.

EXERCISE 7

Identify a support network. A problem for many of us is that we often expect most, or all, of our support to come from our immediate family. Extend your support network so that there is more choice in a crisis and less emotional dependence on one or two people. List different types of support.

➤ Someone I can depend on to give me constructive criticism.
➤ Someone I feel really close to.
➤ Someone who introduces me to new people and ideas.
➤ Someone I enjoy chatting to.
➤ Someone who makes me feel competent and valued.
➤ Someone who is always a valuable source of information.
➤ Someone who will challenge me to sit up and take a good look at myself.
➤ Someone I can depend on in a crisis.
➤ Someone I can share bad news with.
➤ Someone I can share good news and good feelings with.

You may find that your support network will be different for home and work problems.

Once you have compiled the list, you will be able to use friends, colleagues or acquaintances for more than just a sounding board for your circuitous problems. Very rarely does one person provide all the different levels of support equally well.

EXERCISE 8

Learn some basic counselling skills (*see* Chapter 10, Developing interview skills, in Section 3) and then go on to try the following.

1 The stress interview

Ask a friend to 'interview' you by asking leading questions about a stressful experience. They can write down the responses and may prompt you by saying such things as 'Tell me more about that', 'How did you feel then?', 'Is there anything else you want to say about the incident?'.

The friend is not permitted to comment, give advice or criticise – just to give attention and support. He or she may not need to say or do anything but give you time to talk; you will know the answers yourself but just need time to sort them out. The interviewer asks the following questions.

➤ Think about something that happened to you that was a very stressful experience for you. Tell me about it.
➤ Was this something you knew was going to happen or was it a surprise to you?

➤ What did you feel when this happened and what did you do?

➤ Can you remember doing anything that made you feel any better or less anxious? Describe what you did.

➤ Did you turn to anyone else for help?

➤ If you had to face that again, would you do anything different now? Could you have done anything to prevent it happening or that would have made it less stressful for you?

➤ Did you learn anything about yourself as a result of the experience?

2   Co-counsel[35]

Co-counselling is a form of personal or psychological peer counselling in which two or more people alternate the roles of therapist and patient. Originally formulated in the United States, co-counselling is reciprocal peer counselling, where participants take it in equal turns to be client and counsellor. Key to the method is that it is cost-free, each participant is equal, neither party becomes an 'expert', the person being client stays in charge of the session and the person being counsellor mainly just gives very good, non-judgemental and loving attention.

Co-counselling can be used to help us get better at most things and in most ways. It can be used to deal with day-to-day life problems or it can be used to deal with deep personal distress. Co-counselling is a highly effective tool for personal development. Those who have used the method feel that certain qualities mean that co-counsellors move quickly in dealing with their issues. Perhaps because the client is in charge, no one is pushing the client to do anything they do not choose to do, and everything is accepted unconditionally. Co-counsellors develop emotional competence: that is, they become comfortable with emotions and the expression of emotion both in themselves and in others.

To use co-counselling techniques, take some protected time (the boundaries are important, otherwise the session may degenerate into a mutual, ineffective, chat).

Allow 10 or 15 minutes each to begin with, building up to 30 or 45 minute slots. Alternate the roles of 'therapist' and 'patient' in turn to listen to each other without commenting or giving advice. The person being client stays in charge of the session and the person being counsellor uses first-line counselling skills: not counselling or advising but encouraging – mainly non-verbally, giving very good, non-judgemental, listening and loving attention. Allow the 'client' to be completely in charge of their own material, and never push them to do anything that they do not choose to do. Accept all talk and emotions unconditionally.

Through sharing our innermost worlds with others, and risking them seeing our 'darker' side, we develop safe ways of normalising difficult feelings and

---

35 www.co-counselling.org.uk (accessed April 2013).

releasing pent-up emotions. We allow ourselves to accept that emotions have a role in helping us to handle danger, aggression and abandonment more effectively, to have fun and feel more loving. We are able to relate with others more clearly and effectively because we no longer have to avoid, deny or suppress our emotions, but acknowledge and share them more comfortably.

Take in the good

There is a 'negativity bias' to the brain (e.g. it typically takes around five positive interactions to overcome the effects of a single negative one),[36] so it takes an active effort to internalise positive experiences and heal negative ones. Positive feelings have far-reaching benefits, including physical and psychological benefits such as a stronger immune system, a cardiovascular system that is more immune to stress, and they help to counteract the effects of painful experiences – benefits noted by researchers such as Frederickson *et al.*[37] Taking in the good means rebuilding new and necessary neural structures, consolidating these experiences in memory, focusing mindfully on the positive aspects of life and highlighting key states of mind such as kindness and inner peace, so you can find a quick way back to them in times of trouble. It is about nourishing well-being, contentment and the peaceful aspects of ourselves that we can return to when needed. The method can be used in many ways: whenever we experience something positively, allow it to sink into and soothe us to replace old pains; when negative material arises, bring to mind emotions and perspectives that are its antidote;[38] and to develop self-compassion – warmth, concern and good wishes for yourself – which, the Mindfulness literature tells us, helps to build resilience.

Avoiding stress

Can stress be avoided? Avoidance of a stress *situation* as a strategy may be workable, but CBT practitioners tell us that it is not helpful to engage in thoughts and situations you cannot change.[39] If you focus on, allow yourself to be irritated by or, paradoxically, resist the thoughts and feelings about what is happening, your stress levels will rise. It is the endless focus on the past and future – which cannot be changed or predicted – that creates the painful tension and anxiety. If, however, you peacefully and meditatively examine

36 Gottman (1995). Cited in: Hanson R, Mendius R. *Buddha's Brain: the practical neuroscience of happiness, love and wisdom*. New Harbinger Publications; 2009. pp. 41, 75.

37 Frederickson, Levenson, Mancuso, *et al.* (1998, 2000, 2001). Cited in: Hanson R, Mendius R. *Buddha's Brain: the practical neuroscience of happiness, love and wisdom*. New Harbinger Publications; 2009. p. 75.

38 Hanson R, Mendius R. *Buddha's Brain: the practical neuroscience of happiness, love and wisdom*. New Harbinger Publications; 2009. pp. 76–7.

39 Willson R, Branch R. *Cognitive Behaviour Therapy for Dummies*. John Wiley & Sons; 2006.

a difficult thought, accepting and acknowledging it, as recommended by Mindfulness practitioners,[40] this can be a useful strategy. Those who meditate in this way accept thoughts, feelings, sensations, etc. in the moment, without resistance. Through recognising that anxiety, fear, dread and apprehension are mental states like any other, it diffuses the fear of the emotion itself. If you verbally describe to yourself what is happening, and what you are feeling, you increase the frontal lobe's regulation of the limbic system, which is activated in the fear response.[41]

In this next section we look at some of the ways individuals normally deal with perceived threats, that may or may not be stressful, in different ways. There are different classifications for these coping, or defence, mechanisms; however, they all are variations on the same general idea: there are good/productive ways to handle stress, and there are negative/counterproductive ways to do so. Because stress is perceived, the following mechanisms do not necessarily deal with the actual situation that is causing an individual stress. However, they may be considered coping mechanisms if they allow the individual to cope better with the negative feelings/anxiety that they are experiencing due to the perceived stressful situation, as opposed to actually fixing the concrete obstacle causing them stress.

We begin by looking at some of the ways we all manage stress, that may be counter-productive.

Counterproductive ways of dealing with stress: mental inhibitions

We all adopt these processes as they can diminish the awareness of anxiety, threat, fear, etc. that comes when we are conscious of a perceived threat. In mild cases, they are seen as common, unconscious, coping or defence mechanisms which we apply at times to seek to master, minimise or tolerate stress, including boredom or conflict. Such mechanisms are common to us all, but, as can be seen, are not considered useful as they are mental states that are best made conscious, recognised, acknowledged and worked with. One of the most important things that assertiveness can teach us is about understanding ourselves and others better, developing our emotional IQ, so that the following problems do not hold us back in our dealings with ourselves and others.

➤ **Denial:** if we are faced with a fact that is too uncomfortable to accept, it may be rejected, with insistence that it is not true despite what may be overwhelming evidence to the contrary. This may be simple denial (denying the reality of the unpleasant fact altogether), minimisation

---

40 Kabat-Zinn, note 28 above. Alidina, note 28 above.
41 Lieberman, *et al.* (2007). Cited in: Hanson R, Mendius R. *Buddha's Brain: the practical neuroscience of happiness, love and wisdom.* New Harbinger Publications; 2009. p. 90.

(admitting the fact but denying its seriousness) or projection(admitting both the fact and seriousness but denying responsibility).

➤ **Dissociation:**[42] an experience of detachment or loss from one's immediate surroundings and physical and emotional reality.

➤ **Projection:**[43] where a person subconsciously denies his or her own attributes, thoughts and emotions, which are then usually ascribed to other people. This has the effect of reducing anxiety by allowing the expression of the impulses or desires without letting the conscious mind recognise them.

➤ **Rationalisation:**[44] when perceived controversial behaviours or feelings are logically justified and explained in a rational or logical manner in order to avoid any true explanation. They are thus made consciously tolerable – or even admirable and superior – by plausible means.

Other counterproductive methods deal with stress by an individual literally taking action, or withdrawing.

➤ **Acting out:** problematic behaviour. Instead of reflecting or problem solving, an individual takes maladaptive action.[45]

➤ **Passive-aggression:** discussed earlier as a non-assertive response. An individual indirectly deals with his or her anxiety and negative thoughts/ feelings stemming from their stress by acting in a hostile or resentful manner towards others. Manipulative, help-rejecting and complaining behaviours can also be included in this category.

It is useful for us to be aware of any of these traits within us, so that we can name them and own them in our dealings with others. By acknowledging them, we can significantly reduce the stress levels that occur during conflicted conversations.

Here we look at some of the other positive, life-affirming techniques that can be used by each of us in our daily lives to reduce our own stress levels.

Problem solving

These skills are good coping mechanisms that face the problem, dealing with the negative emotions evoked by stress in a constructive, assertive manner.

---

42 Dell PF, O'Neil JA. Preface. In: Dell PF, O'Neil JA, editors. *Dissociation and the Dissociative Disorders: DSM-V and beyond.* Routledge; 2009. pp. xix–xxi.

43 Wade T. *Psychology.* 6th ed. Prentice Hall; 2000.

44 Berne E. *A Layman's Guide to Psychiatry and Psychoanalysis.* Ballantine Books; 1980.

45 Adapted from: American Psychological Association. *DSM-IV Adaptive Functioning Scale.* American Psychological Association; 1994.

➤ **Affiliation:** using a social network for support, sharing ideas with others.[46]

➤ **Humour:** which enables us to gain perspective, to step outside of the situation.[47]

➤ **Sublimation:**[48] channelling troubled emotions or impulses into an outlet that is socially acceptable.

➤ **Positive reappraisal:** refocusing and redirecting thoughts (cognitions) to good things that are either occurring or have not occurred. This can lead to personal growth, self-reflection and awareness of the power/benefits of one's efforts.[49]

➤ **Anticipation:** preparing for the event.

➤ **Self-observation:** to increase emotional intelligence.

➤ **Aerobic exercise:** those who consistently make time for aerobic exercise tend to report reduced stress. Research has shown that aerobic exercises, such as jogging, are associated with improved hormonal responses to stress and a decrease in depressive mood states.[50]

Minimising stress

The following mechanisms are adapted from the DSM-IV Adaptive Functioning Scale[51] and other local references.[52] They are simple techniques that can be applied by the individual themselves as healthy coping mechanisms to minimise stress.

Behavioural and lifestyle changes

➤ Develop physical resilience by eating well and regularly, taking exercise (which counteracts any increased muscular tensions, increases the levels of endorphins, and improves mental and physical health), establishing a good sleep pattern, and looking after your living environment.

➤ Strike a good work/life balance: develop interests outside work and book frequent breaks.

➤ Do not isolate yourself. Your friends and family can provide you with a great deal of energy, affection and emotional support.

---

46 Levo L. Understanding defence mechanisms. *Lukenotes*. 2003; **7**(4). St Luke Institute, MD. And adapted from *DSM-IV Adaptive Functioning Scale*, note 45 above.

47 Levo, note 46 above.

48 Valliant G. Adaptive mental mechanisms. *American Psychologist*. 2000; **55**(1): 89–98. Willson, Branch, note 39 above.

49 Folkman S, Moskowitz J. Stress, positive emotion, and coping. *Current Directions in Psychological Science*. 2000; **9**(4): 115–18.

50 Carlson, Heth, note 14 above, pp. 537–8.

51 *See* note 45 above.

52 NHS Somerset. *The Little Book of Mental Health: a practical guide for everyday emotional wellbeing*. Available at: www.hp.somerset.nhs.uk (accessed April 2013). Saulsman L, Nathan P, Lim L, *et al. What? Me Worry!?! Mastering your worries*. Centre for Clinical Interventions; 2005.

➤ Develop emotional resilience and inner strength: relish your relationships, hold a self-accepting attitude, use humour.
➤ Make sure you are in the right job and, once there, keep up to date, create a good team around you, and be clear that you cannot do everything.
➤ Stay psychologically and emotionally fit: see a counsellor; take a compassionate look at yourself – accepting perspective to reduce any shame or guilt you may feel. Reduce rumination by focussing on the moment, recognise negative thoughts as symptoms not facts.

You can reduce the harmful effects of work stress and protect yourself against future pressures by establishing such an anti-stress lifestyle.

Food too has an important role to play in fighting stress. Mindfulness practitioners believe that how you eat is more important than what you eat when you are under stress. Look at how, what and when you eat. Eat slowly and well. Savour your food. If you are under a great deal of stress or emotional trauma, you are likely to need more of the B-complex vitamins, vitamin C and minerals such as zinc. This also applies to people who smoke, drink alcohol or take antibiotics. It is equally important to avoid using stimulants such as alcohol, coffee or cigarettes. These exacerbate by artificially altering your physiological balance: alcohol is a sedative, not a stimulant. It dulls the memory and concentration, and impairs performance. Women are more likely than men to smoke for negative reasons, believing that it helps to combat anger and anxiety. Initially, the effects are helpful, but a craving that is much stronger than the original stress follows them. Keep on trying to give up: the more you disrupt your habit, the easier it becomes to kick it. Mood swings and emotional outbursts are more common among drinkers. If you are getting heavy hints from friends or relatives, and you cannot cut down, consult your GP.

When you are under stress, relaxation often requires a conscious effort. Tranquillity involves parasympathetic, stress-reductive activation. Develop reflective periods in your self-created hectic life programme. Cultivate a slower pace of living. Do one thing at a time, and concentrate on it, avoiding collecting chores up or multi-tasking, for example, avoid making a phone call and surfing the net simultaneously. Create stress-free breathing spaces during the course of the day, perhaps to do isometric, relaxation or deep-breathing exercises. Try non-competitive exercises that force you to slow down such as yoga, which is a useful anti-stress weapon, being both physically demanding and non-competitive. Meditation is becoming a very popular and evidence-based way of calming or stilling your mind even further than relaxation does. It is a deeper and fuller form of relaxation, so is therefore more fulfilling, and better for you. Choose a form of meditation that suits you: not all methods suit everyone. There are many methods: self-hypnosis, Mindfulness, prayer, Buddhist meditation, guided fantasy, body scanning. If you follow a religion, be proud that you gain strength from your beliefs. Take time out before and after for rest and relaxation or meditation, otherwise you are negating the effect.

While in the office, set an alert periodically to encourage you to stop what you are doing for a couple of minutes and look out of the window: enjoy the respite, a brief period of non-doing. Build in some office or chair-based exercises.

➤ Massage the fingers of each hand in turn.

➤ Rub your scalp with fingertips, concentrating on the hairline.

➤ Place the fingers of both hands on either side of the back of your neck. Press and move them slowly outwards from the centre, breathing deeply.

➤ Eye rolling: start by 'looking' very slowly round your field of vision in a clockwise direction. Repeat anti-clockwise

➤ Close your eyes; stroke them with your fingertips 10 times.

➤ Stand with your legs slightly apart and shake out the tension from your hands and lower arms.

➤ Take a deep breath and exhale slowly. Imagine you are releasing the pent-up energy with every breath out. This is both energising and relaxing, activating both the sympathetic and parasympathetic nervous system.

➤ Roll your head slowly, or hunch your shoulders up towards your neck and then release.

➤ Alternately tense then release muscle groups.

➤ Book an Indian head massage. Some therapists provide a home or work visiting service, which can be an ideal solution for busy workers. Give yourself a quick 'lift' by massaging trouble spots at any time, without the use of lotions. Imagine as you massage that you are dispelling all the tension and energy out from your body into the air around you.

➤ Close your eyes for a few minutes and imagine yourself in a beautiful place. Again, choose a place that is right for you: it may be a hot, sunny beach, it may be a cool moonlit night, it may be a grassy riverbank. Take yourself on a journey through your imagination and see what happens.

Cognitive changes that aid decision making

Much of the work of CBT therapists and life goal coaches is to encourage us to become smarter and more proactive in taking charge of and managing our lives. These cognitive and behavioural changes can help to reduce stress levels. When pressures are allowed to get out of hand, you become less able to deal efficiently with the problems that face you. Take yourself away from the problem and then you can deal with it. Some simple changes may be to:

➤ deal immediately with any external event that causes stress, such as harassment or bullying at work – do not procrastinate

➤ programme yourself for change – sign on for a meditation class, take up karate

➤ give yourself some constructive self-talk or 'positive affirmations' ('I am good at my job/a good parent/have a good sense of humour') – say these aloud, regularly

➤ change some attitudes – you may not be able to change other peoples' behaviour, but you can change your own reaction to it

➤ learn to deflect irritating behaviours, simply by choosing to ignore them

➤ brainstorm solutions to your stress problems

➤ schedule activities, so gradually introducing reinforcement back into your life.

Be active in choosing and achieving the goals: make them specific, positive ('I want to be more assertive' rather than 'I want to be less passive'), observable (how would other people notice that the goal had been achieved?), realistic (within your reach and control); goals that involve changing yourself not others, and timely – within a timeframe to enable you to remain focused and motivated.

Another technique is to get the thoughts out of our head and onto paper, so changing them to another, more manageable form.

➤ Make use of hierarchies, lists and *grids* to identify positive and negative thoughts, behaviours, options. Identify and weight pros and cons. Take time over this, as decision making itself can cause stress: the choice may be between two equally attractive options (the approach-approach conflict); two equally unattractive options (avoidance-avoidance conflict); or something that has both attractive and unattractive traits, such as whether to attend university or take a gap year – here the decisions around loans/employment/friendships make this an complex conflict.

➤ Use ranking to make your choices clearer when making decisions. Identify the problem (you want to change jobs but cannot make that first move). List, on one side of the page, the reasons for wanting to change; on the other side, list the reasons why you cannot change. Give each reason a numerical weighting, then total up the scores.

CBT therapists use cognitive reframing to challenge any destructive self-talk, as described above in relation to the Type B personalities. Here, we challenge any destructive beliefs, where we set impossibly high targets for ourselves that are impossible to attain, with logic. Common destructive beliefs are around perfectionism and uncertainty.

> Destructive: 'Disagreement and conflict are a disaster and must be avoided at all costs.'
>
> versus
>
> Constructive: 'I can learn from conflicts. It is possible to disagree and still remain friends.'

Destructive: 'I must be perfect.'

versus

Constructive: 'Perfection is impossible to attain. The world is not perfect, nor can we be.'

Other ways to challenge negative behaviour patterns include moderating your stress. Find out how vulnerable you are to stress, then tackle it by modifying your behaviour. If you find this hard, begin by moderating your own self-induced stress.

➤ Get organised.
➤ Try to limit any behaviour that you recognise as being obsessional or time-dominated. If you cannot, seek professional help.
➤ Do not set unrealistic deadlines.
➤ Learn to differentiate between urgent tasks and less important aspects of your work.
➤ Not everything requires immediate action. Much more important is the quality of the results.
➤ Try to restrain yourself from having to be the centre of attention by constantly talking: force yourself really to listen to others.
➤ Avoid being too work-orientated.
➤ Schedule some non-competitive activities into your leisure time. If you take up a competitive sport such as squash, trying to beat an opponent is just as bad in stress terms as trying to beat a work colleague.
➤ Learn to enjoy things, rather than treating them simply as a means to an end.
➤ Learn to laugh more, be lighter on yourself.
➤ In any discussion, do not be on the offensive – you are out to talk, not to do battle. Use a balance of logic, assertiveness and good humour.

Improving long-term survival states

Ancient philosophy, Buddhist wisdom, modern cognitive behavioural therapy and Mindfulness methods are advocated to help to relax the self and lead a happy life. By working to develop, and adopting, fundamental principles and values that promote feelings of kindness, compassion, humility, virtue, benevolence, openness, wisdom and generosity towards self and others,[53] we help ourselves to maintain a strong, relaxed sense of self. It is through the connection with others that we learn to reduce our dependency on our own ego, which is that which makes us feel special, but also disconnects us from, and puts us in opposition with, others, negating any feelings of peace,

---

53 Hanson, Mendius, note 38 above, pp. 215–19, 76–7.

contentment and connectedness. It is helpful to relax about what others think, renounce the need constantly to seek approval. It is hard to release negative states of mind such as pride, envy and jealousy, but it is worth considering what these feelings create in us. The Mindfulness literature reminds us not to resist the feelings if they arise, but to note them and move on: not to resist any feelings or situations but be awake and open to their happening. Through this we may obtain, if not happiness, a reduction in fear and anxiety and a sense of calm, to be at peace with ourselves.

It is not easy to work at changing a life stance, a belief set, but it is through developing a different sense of the world, and our position in it, that we begin to open to the possibility of a less stressful, personally fulfilling existence.

A core principle is if we understand that, despite our best wishes, everything keeps changing, everything is connected, opportunities routinely remain unfulfilled, and many threats are inescapable (e.g. aging and death), we begin to accept uncertainty. Even our sense of self is impermanent, as our physical and mental selves are continually in the process of change, being constructed and deconstructed, never static. This is a difficult cognitive shift, given that we humans have developed certain useful strategies for survival: the creation of boundaries, to separate ourselves from the world and one internal state from the other; the maintenance of stability (physical and mental systems in balance); and the need to approach opportunities and avoid threats.[54] But it is through understanding that fundamentally all life is uncertain that we have a good chance of managing the stresses it throws our way.

Significant trauma

It is not the place of this book to discuss entrenched or significant trauma and its sequelae, but it is worth noting that if you are aware of events in your life that trigger more complex and painful feelings, take charge and look for professional help. When a traumatic experience occurs, it may overwhelm usual cognitive and neurological coping mechanisms, the memory and associated stimuli of the event are inadequately processed, and are stored in an isolated memory network. The goal of psychological therapy is to allow clients to process these distressing memories, reducing their lingering influence and allowing them to develop more adaptive coping mechanisms.[55] It is assertive to acknowledge

---

54 Hanson, Mendius, note 38 above, p. 26.
55 Australian Centre for Posttraumatic Mental Health. *Australian Guidelines for the Treatment of Adults with Acute Stress Disorder and Post Traumatic Stress Disorder.* Australian Centre for Posttraumatic Mental Health; 2007. Foa EB, Keane TM, Friedman MJ. *Effective Treatments for PTST: practice guidelines of the International Society for Traumatic Stress Studies.* The Guilford Press; 2009. Herbert J, Lilienfeld S, Lohr J, *et al.* Science and pseudoscience in the development of eye movement desensitization and reprocessing: implications for clinical psychology. *Clinical Psychology Review.* 2000; **20**(8): 945–71.

that at times in life we may have difficulty managing our stresses alone, and be open to accepting professional help.

Some of the statistics on stress are disturbing. It is commonly known that at least one in 10 people in the UK will spend some time in secondary mental health care at least once in their life. Work-related stress is defined as a harmful reaction people have to undue pressures and demands place on them at work. The latest estimates from the Labour Force Survey show that although the total number of new cases of stress for work-related illnesses in 2010/11 was significantly lower than the number in 2001/02, the industries that reported the highest rates of work-related stress in the last three years were health, social work, education and public administration, in particular, health and social service managers, teachers and social welfare associate professionals. Many of us are threatening our physical and mental well-being by approaching 'burn out', a phrase that describes an overdose of stress factors perfectly. Burn out, and the symptoms of stress, are reversible. The sooner we start being kinder to ourselves, and teaching our patients and clients to be kind to themselves, the better.

In the light of this, it may be worth considering the following orders for a stress-free life.[56]

> ➤ Thou shalt not try to be all things to all people.
> ➤ Thou shalt not be perfect or even try.
> ➤ Thou shalt leave undone things that ought to be done.
> ➤ Thou shalt not spread thyself too thin.
> ➤ Thou shalt learn to say 'no'.
> ➤ Thou shalt schedule time for thyself and thy supportive network.
> ➤ Thou shalt switch off and do nothing regularly.
> ➤ Thou shalt be boring, inelegant, untidy and unattractive at times.
> ➤ Thou shalt not feel guilty.
> ➤ Thou shalt not be thine own worst enemy.

Assertion as a stress buster

Behaving assertively is a massive step towards reducing stress levels, inner negative self-talk and rumination.

➤ Tackle relationship problems and communication breakdowns at source. Is it lack of time? Poor communication? Deal with the problem assertively.
➤ Put aside time from all your other activities to give to yourself, regularly.
➤ Be open about your feelings, especially anger or fear.
➤ Be assertive: ask for what you want, and learn how to say 'no'.

---

56 Edmondson C. *Minister: love thyself! – sustaining healthy ministry (pastoral)*. Grove Books; 2000.

KEY POINTS

➤ Stress is a pattern of physiological, behavioural, emotional and cognitive responses to real or imagined stimuli. Thus external stressors have different effects on different people, and stress is a personal perception and response, the resilience to which is based on personality and skills, which can be learned and developed.

➤ Stress needs to be part of everyday life, as it helps keep us alert and out of danger. In small doses, it can create a 'high' where challenges are enjoyed, and it accounts for feelings of excitement and optimism when a new venture is started.

➤ The physiological responses to stress demand much of the body's energy and resources, and have a great impact on disease and risk for disease. Our bodies cannot tell the difference between events that are actual threats to survival and events that are present in thoughts alone.

➤ There are said to be three stress categories: crises/catastrophes; major life events; and daily hassles/micro-stressors, which includes the most commonly occurring type of stressor in everyday life. Physiologically, day-to-day/chronic stressors have a greater negative impact on individuals' health than do more acute, traumatic stressors.

➤ Some of the most common forms of stress at work have been identified as relationship stresses, intrinsic to the job role, work under- or overload, problems with rules and regulations and the home/work balance. Decision making itself can cause stress.

➤ When risk-assessing to see how stressed we are, another way of analysing our propensity to stress is to look at four variables: the demands on our life; our relationships; the level of control we have; and our support systems. Stress is exacerbated when we have a taste of power but cannot wield much influence, and when we work in a climate of uncertainty, chaos and the unknown.

➤ There are personality differences. Those who tend to work in fast-moving jobs that require an extrovert personality and also quick decision-making may chose to manage in an environment of rapid change and development. In the struggle to achieve more in less time, it is often at the expense of others, and even your own health. Less extreme, quieter, more passive personalities may need to challenge destructive self-talk through cognitive reframing techniques. More moderate or passive personalities may benefit from talking more about their feelings.

➤ Some of the supporting approaches used in developing resilience are in developing confidence, adaptability, purposefulness and social support; therapeutic techniques such as problem solving skills, behavioural and lifestyle changes. What helps is the ability to maintain a sense of humour, flexibility, optimism, seeing challenges as opportunities.

➤ Through sharing our innermost worlds with others, and risking them seeing our 'darker' side, we develop safe ways of normalising difficult feelings. We are able to relate with others more clearly and effectively because we no longer have to avoid, deny or suppress our emotions, but instead acknowledge and share them more comfortably.

➤ It helps to internalise positive experiences and heal negative ones. Focus mindfully on the positive aspects of life, highlighting key states of mind such as kindness and inner peace, so that you can find a quick way back to them in times of trouble. Develop self-compassion – warmth, concern and good wishes for yourself. It is not helpful to engage in thoughts and situations that you cannot change. Peacefully and meditatively examine a difficult thought, accept and acknowledge it.

➤ There are good/productive ways to handle stress, and there are negative/counterproductive ways to do so, through denial, dissociation, projection, rationalisation and acting out.

➤ Minimise stress through simple cognitive and behavioural and lifestyle changes: programme yourself for change; strike a good work/life balance, eating, drinking, sleeping and exercising moderately; relish relationships. Rest, relax, meditate. Moderate your own self-induced stress through controlling any behaviour that you recognise as being obsessional or time-dominated, learn to enjoy things, rather than treating them simply as a means to an end. Learn to laugh more, be lighter on yourself.

➤ Behaving assertively helps to reduce stress levels, inner negative self-talk and rumination.

➤ Develop the values that promote feelings of kindness, compassion, humility, virtue, benevolence, openness, wisdom and generosity towards self and others that help us to develop connections with ourselves and others. Through this we may obtain a sense of calm, to be at peace with ourselves.

FURTHER READING

Alindina S. *Mindfulness for Dummies*. John Wiley & Sons; 2010.

Birnbaum L, Birnbaum A. Mindful social work: from theory to practice. *Journal of Religion & Spirituality in Social Work*. 2008; **27**: 87–104.

British Heart Foundation. *Coping with Stress: how to manage stress and help your heart*. British Heart Foundation; 2010. Available at: www.bhf.org.uk/publications (accessed April 2013).

Burkeman O. At: www.actionforhappiness.org/ (accessed April 2013).

Crane RC, Kyken W. The implementation of Mindfulness-based cognitive therapy: learning from the UK health service experience. *Mindfulness*. Advance publication accessed online at: www.bangor.ac.uk/mindfulness/nhs/php.en (accessed May 2013).

Freudenberger HJ. *Burn Out – how to beat the high cost of success*. Bantam Books; 1980.

Gilbert P. *Mindfulness and Social Work* by Stephen F Hick (ed.), Lyceum Books, 2009 [book review]. *Community Care*. 2010. Available at: www.communitycare.co.uk/Articles/06/09/2010/115258/book-review-mindfulness-and-social-work.htm (accessed May 2013).

Hanson R, Mendius R. *Buddha's Brain: the practical neuroscience of happiness, love and wisdom*. New Harbinger Publications; 2009.

Hick S, editor. *Mindfulness and Social Work*. Lyceum Books; 2009.

Kabat-Zinn J. *Full Catastrophe Living: how to cope with stress, pain and illness using Mindfulness meditation*. Piatkus; 2001.

Kenny MA, Williams JMG. Treatment resistant depressed patients show a good response to Mindfulness-based cognitive therapy. *Behaviour Research and Therapy*. 2007; **45**: 617–25.

Kuyken W, Byford S, Taylor LR, *et al*. Mindfulness-based cognitive therapy to prevent relapse in recurrent depression. *Journal of Consulting and Clinical Psychology*. 2008; **76**: 966–78.

National Institute for Health and Clinical Excellence. *Depression in Adults: the treatment and management of depression in adults: NICE guideline 90* [partial update of *NICE guideline 23*]. NIHCE; 2009. www.nice.org.uk/CG90fullguideline (accessed May 2013).

Ready R, Burton K. *Neurolinguistic Programming for Dummies*. John Wiley & Sons; 2010.

Segal ZJ, Williams MG, Teasdale JD. *Mindfulness-based Cognitive Therapy for Depression: a new approach to preventing relapses*. The Guilford Press; 2002.

Tolle E. *The Power of Now: a guide to spiritual enlightenment*. Hodder and Stoughton; 2005.

Williams M, Penman D. *Mindfulness. A practical guide to finding peace in a frantic world*. Piatkus; 2011.

Willson R, Branch R. *Cognitive Behaviour Therapy for Dummies*. John Wiley & Sons; 2006.

CHAPTER 14

Time management

'It's not enough to be busy. The question is: What are we busy about?'

Henry Thoreau

All of us should build rest and relaxation into our working day to keep us sane and effective, but the pace of work, in the NHS in particular, is such that this is not always possible. Time is a precious resource. In this chapter, we identify who and what wastes our time, and look at some of the ways in which we can use assertiveness to manage these intrusions and build our resilience for a healthier and happier life.

MANAGING TIME

If we feel constantly stressed, one key solution is to learn to control events rather than let them control us. Take charge, plan your work, and you will immediately feel less stressed. Proper organisation gives us a sense of direction and control. When we allow the situation to control us, we follow external and imposed schedules, so we struggle with stress, interruptions, paperwork and procrastination while yearning for freedom and flexibility.

Some time managers believe that many of us spend as much as 80% of our time on non-essential tasks. There are ways of improving our use of time, which will release us to do those important tasks. Here are some ideas to help us take better control of time.

Time stealers[1]

Time is a resource that needs protecting. People who 'steal' time are not usually ill-intentioned. Their demands may inadvertently waste our time: they may talk about situations or events unconnected with our own agenda, or they may distract us with an activity that may be welcomed at a different time, such as gossip. Team working is dependent on good relationships, and these good

---

1   Wynne-Jones M. Time stealers. *Pulse*. 2001; **21**: 4.

relationships do take time to foster and develop, but the key to managing our time is to be in charge of it.

It is up to us to decide, and negotiate, when, where and for how long such conversations take place. If stretched for time and our talking partner is oblivious, make good use of body language: remain standing while you talk, and usher the speaker out by opening the door to indicate their exit. Use paperwork to move the task on, draw attention to the next agenda item, shuffle papers. Or verbalise assertively, take charge: make it clear that the visit/meeting is over: 'Before we finish, I would …' Tell people at the beginning of the meeting how much time you have allocated to it. If you feel you are going to ramble, schedule your meetings before appointments, and get in the habit of using definite times/meetings for discussing routine matters with others. To save on travelling time, try to allocate meetings fairly so that everyone has a chance to meet in their own office.

The following exercise helps us begin to gain control through identifying our own needs.

EXERCISE 1

Make a list of all the things you consider time-wasting activities at work

_____

_____

_____

_____

_____

_____

_____

_____

Manage interruptions

Give clear messages to those who interrupt. Your time – all our time – is expensive. Model this to your colleagues. Give people who offer you information a chance to indicate whether it is urgent; schedule in a good time to hear it. If not, offer a choice: 'I can only spare about a minute now – can it wait?' _Or_ develop 'screening' plans: insist on appointments. Decide which situations colleagues may interrupt you and which things can be postponed, then work quietly in your room with the door shut and the phone diverted. When very stretched for time, you and your team could employ a 'flag' system, where an amount of time each day is designated during which employees agree not to interrupt each other. Use a flag system on the desk: red for 'Do not disturb', orange for 'Come in, but it had better be important', green for availability.

Try standing up when people enter your room. To protect yourself further do not keep a chair near your desk, or designate a clear seating area for one to one meetings. Both of you will be more likely to stay on target. Or meet people at *their* desks when you need something from them. By doing this, you are in control of the visit, and it is easier for you to exit.

Technology

Using phones can be a massive time waster, which is one of the reasons why email has superseded their use so effectively. There are ways of managing time better on the phone, however. To save everyone time, be organised. Always identify self/department/organisation when answering, have a pen and paper by all phones, and do not be kept waiting with an engaged tone – get them to call you back or use a hands-free phone. If on a phone rota, arrange with co-workers to sign up for certain hours during which one of you will answer the phone for everyone. This gives everyone a bit of protected time. If possible, prioritise the time of the most expensive worker and delegate: use your secretary/operator/voice mail to screen calls.

Create telephone protocols so that everyone can take appropriate responsibility for messages, and have a template for taking messages (date, time, who called, who the message is for, number to call back). Avoid engaging with the content of the message (if you cannot help) by asking the caller to return their call or telling them the call will be returned. Delegate, disengage with anything you cannot specifically help the caller with, for example, if the caller asks a clinician the directions to a clinic, promise them a map in the post or pass them on to administrative help.

Plan ahead: list what you want to discuss. It saves time for everybody and makes better communication. Never let yourself be interrupted from the task at hand by a ringing phone: when you take the calls as they come, you allow your work to be randomly disrupted. If you know you tend to waffle, try buying a three-minute sandglass and put it by your phone. See if you can successfully complete every call in three minutes. At work, you need to use the phone to inform, not to chat. Think 'green': ring people instead of writing them letters; phone conference or Skype instead of meeting; use email in preference to the phone for giving information.

Make your technology work for you and utilise all short cuts: use your address books and create easy access systems for numbers/sites used regularly.

Make ample use of computerised diaries that everybody can view, but not edit, to reduce the need for paperwork and memos. Think first: what is the quickest/safest/best way to communicate this: email rather than snail mail? Write instead of phoning? Phone instead of visiting?

Report writing

The first consideration when writing letters and reports is to know the reader and purpose. Use the four-step method (prepare, arrange, write, revise), keeping it short and simple, avoiding jargon. Turn weekly reports into monthly reports and monthly reports into quarterly reports. Try to keep to one document: a care plan instead of a report, a report instead of a letter – are you duplicating unnecessarily?

Crisis management

Learn to say 'no'! Do one job at a time, and do it well. Drop old responsibilities when you accept new ones, and always consider whether you have set yourself too high a task or too many objectives to manage. Ignore anything of minor importance which is going to hold you up. Delegate those tasks that your subordinates can handle.

Paper chain

Common irritants in general practice have been identified as:
➤ lost papers
➤ illegible cryptic scrawls
➤ incorrect or incomplete facts
➤ delays in processing paperwork
➤ failure to follow agreed practice systems or protocols.[2]

Each time a task is not properly completed, the next person involved in the work has an additional burden. Ultimately, all the paperwork in healthcare relates to client care, and while one member of the team may sometimes be indifferent, others are not, and they may feel compelled to complete the work properly so that the patient does not suffer. It should be the responsibility of everybody – including the clinicians – to ensure that their part of the chain of work is completed in a proper and timely fashion: no short cuts (if these are possible, the system is plainly wrong), no putting on one side and forgetting, no avoiding the system – it was put in place for a reason.

Everyone should be able to rely on their team workers, and expect them to turn round the paperwork reliably, legibly and accurately. Make it clear that a disorganised approach is not tolerated: in the working world there is an

---

2 Hawksley N. Paper chase. *Practice Manager.* 2000; **8**: 21–2.

inherent expectation that people should be organised and look after important paperwork and equipment, and managers should be able to manage their staff so to receive a consistent response and behaviour from each one. To achieve this, managers should act like managers, and clinicians like clinicians, and delegate reception or secretarial duties. Highly skilled and highly paid people within the team should be discouraged from doing jobs that someone less qualified can do for less. To this end, introduce systems for note tracing, message taking and appointments. Improve communication, become better organised, and keep the setting clean and tidy. A messy and untidy workplace is disruptive and inefficient. People will have to disrupt and interrupt each other to ask where things are. Make liberal use of protocols and schedules so the system runs efficiently.

Administration

Analyse *why* you avoid processing paperwork. Does it bore you or is it difficult? If you find it hard to deal with paperwork and you are a naturally messy worker, do not be responsible for cluttering up other people's desks and lives, and avoid scraps of paper for making notes. Have only one item you are working on in view at a time. Try to designate one of the lower drawers of your desk as a 'dump' drawer. Into this drawer will go all low-priority items such as routine reports, brochures, newspaper cuttings and other pieces which are not urgent. Let these items 'ripen' for a month, then throw them away. Throw away anything about things you cannot influence and which do not affect your working life: immediately delete junk emails and faxes, then sort correspondence into logical priority order and delegate the routine correspondence to others.

If you struggle with paper mountains, and need to keep track of who has read important documents, think about how often do you handle paper. Put a small dot in the upper corner of each piece every time you pick it up to read. Handle each piece of paper once and then act: file, shred or bin. If action is required, write notes in the margin, in pencil, with a clear short sentence. Annotate as it passes round the team, with each person initialling their contribution. If a deadline is clearly marked on a letter, ask everyone to add the date they dealt with it. (This not only instils a sense of urgency, but also highlights who is sitting on letters and who is dealing with them promptly.)

If you need help to organise yourself, use either paper systems or technology. There are many computer applications that are designed to help you keep notes, appointments, a diary or calendar. If you prefer a paper-based system, keep a file to remind you of forthcoming deadlines, important things to do and projects to follow up. The system has two major divisions: the first is a set of 12 file folders (one for each month of the year), and the second is *one* set of folders for each day of the month. The current month is placed first in the drawer with the days behind it. Prioritise them.

Other useful, and tried and tested, systems are to date-stamp all documents arriving in the organisation, using a post book to record all incoming and outgoing mail, and leaving letters unsealed until the post is ready to be franked and posted so that the sender can retrieve or add to the contents if necessary.

Speed read

To save time, speed read each section heading of a document, previewing each section, before you read the whole, then read and relate the details to the overall theme. This strategy improves both your comprehension and your recall. Take a moment to practise this on a book: with your hand in a relaxed position, sweep it down the middle of the pages. Do not go all the way to either margin, but stop about a quarter of an inch short of the print on each side of the page. Allow the movement of your hand to guide your eyes smoothly down the page. Do not force your eyes to follow your hand exactly; instead let them drift back and forth looking for ideas.

Take charge of and organise your time so you allocate a specific time for reading: use the daytime to meet people and the early morning, lunchtime or evening to read. Try swapping reading. Set the agenda assertively and be proactive with your ideas. Perhaps arrange for a colleague to read certain articles or journals and you to read others, or lunch together to exchange information and cuttings. Recognise that more can be less: ominous-looking volumes often are not as long as they appear, so only read what you need to in order to understand the main point: the abstract or summary of journals, for example.

Delegate

Remember to delegate anything someone can do *better*, *quicker*, *cheaper* than, or *instead* of, you, but not confidential matters, legally/contractually restricted jobs, disciplinary actions or ultimate accountability.

Manage meetings

Well-planned and managed meetings are an organisation's most valuable means of communication – they considerably ease the task of co-ordinating the activities of large and diverse organisations like the health service. Note whether your meetings are well chaired, organised or not, have good attendance, are held frequently enough, or if there is an absence of relevant supporting paperwork. Although most people do not like meetings, they are unfortunately essential to foster good two-way communication, and need to be held regularly. Senior managers and clinicians demonstrate their commitment to their employees through attending meetings. Staff need to feel included in the major decision making, they need to have ownership of the process.

Dr Vivien Martin discusses some common themes to managing unproductive meetings, which she attributes to ineffective control – of people and time.[3] Here are some of her suggestions.

➤ The chair must demonstrate control of the meeting.
➤ Interrupt and move unproductive time-wasters or hecklers on to something else.
➤ Use a skilled, firm and authoritative chair. Interrupt people who begin philosophical discussions or tell long-winded jokes or anecdotes.
➤ Summarise and restate if people are inarticulate or rambling, or simply glance obtrusively at your watch.
➤ Manage personality clashes as these can factionalise your group and severely hamper discussion:
  – draw attention back to the point of the meeting
  – cut across the argument with direct questions on the topic
  – restate group boundaries: 'We need to keep personalities and judgements out of the discussion'
  – reiterate the objective of the discussion and the time pressures on the meeting.
➤ Point out the constraints under which everyone is operating.
➤ Suggest that they discuss the problem with you privately or raise the issue in a more appropriate forum.
➤ Rehearse or replay meetings without reference to the agenda or minutes
➤ Prevent side conversation.

Meetings often contract (or expand) to fill the time allotted, so shorten them.

Meetings need to be tightly and assertively managed: give incentives to stay on target, try meeting at a different time of day. Review the frequency and duration regularly, and start and finish on time: never delay the meeting for latecomers. Postpone or delegate topics that need further discussion or research. Managers can ensure that action minutes are produced, with name and deadline, and that housekeeping and minute-taking responsibilities are delegated.

We can learn to become more productive ourselves in meetings. We can ask, 'Why are we meeting?' – if an agenda cannot be produced, there is no meeting. We can only speak if we have a real contribution to make, and avoid all meetings that do not run smoothly and productively.

Deal with lateness. Take these tips from MacErlean.[4]

➤ **Calculate the cost of lateness.** If you have 20 people attending a meeting which starts 10 minutes late, your organisation has lost the equivalent of half a day's work.

---

3 Martin V. Meetings management. *Practice Manager*. 2001; **12**: 1.
4 MacErlean N. How to cope with late colleagues. *Observer*. 2001 Aug 19.

➤ **Interrupt lateness:** it shows a strong contempt for people and lack of respect for their time. Bad timekeepers are usually bad administrators – poor at making decisions, unable to say 'no', incapable of critical path analysis and bad at setting priorities. Try to establish a sharper routine.

➤ **Be prompt.** If you let meetings begin late, you are penalising those who have arrived promptly. Never recap for latecomers, but, if desperate, start meetings with the least important item. Try to deal separately with latecomers. Give space for punctual colleagues to air their opinion:

> 'Would anyone like to comment on our timing? Some people were unfortunately delayed – but is there a way we can synchronise watches better in future?'

➤ Never keep people waiting as a way of showing how important you are. This could backfire. Be aware that others may manipulate you in this way, and if so, expose the manipulation by using the assertive questioning techniques set out in Chapter 3, How to be assertive.

Be assertive

If you still passively accept poor delegation, incomplete instructions, too many projects at a time, unclear deadlines, you need to become more assertive about managing yourself and other people. Success at working less and accomplishing more depends on knowing what *not* to do. Over-commitment is one of the most frequent ways we dilute our effectiveness.

➤ Be selective. Learn to say 'no'. Never say 'yes' when you know you could be putting that time to better use.

➤ Ask: 'Am I the right person for this task?'

➤ Do not procrastinate. Answers such as 'I don't know' or 'Let me think about it' only raise false hopes. You have the right to say 'no', and you do not have to offer a reason every time.

➤ Clarify how much authority you have on assignments, then you can continue without constant approval.

➤ Repeat directions in your own words so you are both certain that you have understood the assignment correctly.

Psychologists encourage us to distinguish between urgency and importance.[5] Note that fixing a flat tyre when you are late for an appointment is a matter of great urgency, but its importance is, in most cases, relatively small. Many of us spend our lives fixing flat tyres and ignoring less urgent but more important

---

5   Dickson A. *A Woman in Your Own Right: assertiveness and you*. Revised 30th anniversary ed. Quartet Books; 2012.

matters. In many situations, 20% of what you do yields 80% of your results. Concentrate on those high-payoff items. Of the remaining items:

➤ ask yourself what is the least work that you can do on these and still reach an acceptable standard

➤ then determine which activities you can delegate, which require your limited thought, and which demand your careful attention.

When you are faced with a number of problems, ask yourself which are the truly important ones, and make them your first priority. If you allow yourself to be governed by what is urgent, your life will be one crisis after another. A little foresight, taking steps to prevent potential problems, may ensure that you spend your time achieving your goals rather than reacting to crises.

Work on your emotions

Of all emotions over not getting more done, guilt is one of the most useless. Regret, remorse and bad feeling cannot change the past and they make it difficult to get anything done in the present. Mark Twain once wisely said: 'I have known a great many troubles, but most of them never happened.' Worry, which is future-oriented, is a useless emotion. Follow approaches set by cognitive behaviour therapy and Mindfulness practitioners,[6] and keep in the present. Confront your concern head on. Ask yourself: 'What's the *worst* that could come from this?' When you answer that question, the need for worry usually vanishes.

➤ Replace negative thought patterns. Replace 'What if X happens?' with 'If X happens, I will deal with it by Y'.

➤ If you imagine a catastrophic event, say to yourself: 'And *then* I would [do X] …'

➤ Replace worrying with action planning. Set yourself meaningful goals and go after them. You will soon get so absorbed in their pursuit that you will not have time for worrying.

Ridding yourself of negative emotions can make you a new person. You will find you have time, energy and abilities you never dreamed you had.

Establish your patterns of work

How do you spend your time? If you wish to improve their time management, the starting point is to establish how time is currently used. Keeping a 'time

---

6 Kabat-Zinn J. *Full Catastrophe Living: how to cope with stress, pain and illness using Mindfulness meditation.* Piatkus; 2001. Willson R, Branch R. *Cognitive Behaviour Therapy for Dummies.* John Wiley & Sons; 2006.

diary' can be useful in clarifying not only *how* you spend your time, but also in identifying *who* influences your use of time.

EXERCISE 2

Using a time log

1 Using the form below, record everything you do at work for two to three days. Every minute should be accounted for, and you should be as honest as possible. Make a note of each and every time you change your activity – do not leave it until the end of the day – memory distorts time.

2 Record:
   ➤ the time
   ➤ the activity
   ➤ who initiated the activity (yourself, your staff, a patient, a colleague, external colleagues, etc.)
   ➤ time taken
   ➤ any interruptions (if these are time-consuming they would become activities in their own right).

Daily time log and analysis

Sheet no _____   Today's priorities:

Name   _____   1 _____

Date   _____   2 _____

                                                  3 _____

Time of day	Activity	Who initiated?	Time taken (mins)	Interruptions	Comment critical

Time worked: _____ hours _____ minutes

Keep a diary record of:

(a) content of work

(b) contacts

(c) work priorities

(d) vital tasks.

Set a meeting with yourself at the end of the day to review your daily objectives and set future ones.

EXERCISE 3

Time wasters analysis

Log the time you spend on each time waster.

Time waster	Mon	Tue	Wed	Thu	Fri	Sat	Sun	Total
Unexpected visitors								
Inability to say 'no'								
Trying to do too much at once, and underestimating time required to do the task								
Phone interruptions								
Coffee/tea breaks								
Personal disorganisation								
Indecision on what to do								
Fatigue								
Crisis situations for which no plans were possible								
Wrong information about meeting place, etc.								
Watching television								

Eliminate time wasters

Time waster	Possible causes	Solutions	How you will apply the solutions

EXERCISE 4

List your priorities in terms of work and personal life, giving each a set of goals that you would like to achieve and strategies for achieving them. For example:

Monday

➤ Write up report.
➤ Set up meeting with C.
➤ Send invoices to accounts department.
➤ Phone GP A.
➤ Write and distribute agenda re: team meeting.
➤ Arrange lunch with X.
➤ Check Y ordered new stationery.

If you find that your morning is taken up entirely with the phone calls, so that by lunchtime you have not even considered the report, then your strategy is not working. Ask yourself why – and vow in future to concentrate first on the two priority items, before dealing with the remainder, in order.

Do not make the mistake of working so hard to meet your goals that your life becomes imbalanced, or impose too much routine in your daily schedule so that it becomes monotonous: there is a limit on the time we spend being effective at work.

More time management tips

➤ Avoid taking work home unless you are certain you will do it. Better still, stay for an extra half hour, finish the job and give the evening to your life outside work.
➤ Do jobs requiring mental effort when you are at your best. You may find that in the morning your ideas are good, but you have trouble getting them on paper, and early afternoon is your period of highest writing productivity. So, think about the topics you want to cover in the morning and jot down ideas and put them aside until early afternoon, when you write them out fully.
➤ Set up a fixed daily routine. Schedule definite times for routine matters such as meetings, going through the mail, communicating with your administrative team, signing letters, etc.
➤ Fix deadlines for all jobs. Stick to them.
➤ Do not postpone important matters that are unpleasant. They will block your brain and reduce your creativity and working capacity. Tasks rarely get more pleasant by being postponed.
➤ Put off everything that is not important. Many problems solve themselves if you ignore them for a while.
➤ Hold meetings with yourself. Put a 'Please do not disturb' sign on your

door, with a note showing when you are available. Ask your personal assistant or a colleague to take care of any visitors or telephone calls. Tell the others in the team when you are not available and tell them exactly when they can get hold of you again. And be there.

➤ Do one thing at a time. Keep an overview of the next jobs.

➤ Collect all your ideas in one place: write down the ideas the moment you get them. Go through your ideas regularly and act on them.

➤ When you start a piece of work, finish it. If you split it up too much, you lose track of its coherence, lose your overview and waste your time 'warming up' each time you start again.

➤ Arrange your breaks at times when you cannot work effectively. For instance, when the people you have to talk with are not available, when the material you need is not ready, etc.

➤ Never do anything that you are able to delegate or ignore.

➤ Categorise tasks as important or unimportant, urgent or non-urgent:
1   simple, short-term tasks
2   simple, long-term tasks
3   complex, short-term tasks
4   complex, long-term tasks.

Then do them in the following order:

	Important	Unimportant
Urgent	Do first	Delegate
Non-urgent	Do next	Ignore

Plan your day
➤ Get in the habit of writing a 'to-do' list every day.

➤ Be realistic and aware of the limitations of your time: you can fit in only so many activities. You will feel much better when you finish 10/10 tasks, rather than aiming for but not achieving 20/20.

➤ Plan for the unexpected, such as people being a bit late for appointments.

Organise yourself
➤ Tell yourself that you will work for just 10 minutes. After that, you may have begun to get some sort of a momentum and will not want to stop. If you do stop for some reason, you will be 10 minutes closer to your goal.

➤ Make it a game to finish in time. Cut off your escape. Put away tempting directions.

➤ Work to natural stopping places. You will feel less scattered and more satisfied. For example, do not stop reading in the middle of a section. Finish fully.

➤ If it is your responsibility, deal with big problems yourself immediately – instead of waiting for somebody else to sort it out

➤ Start, no matter what, *start*! If you have a phone call to make, pick up the receiver and start dialling. If you have a letter to write, start typing.

➤ Put time committed to routine daily essentials to a second use: record lecture notes and play them back while dressing or driving, use waiting time to plan, keep the theory notes on hand to read.

➤ Many of us perform some or all of our work at a desk. A desk is a tool that aids in the processing of information, *not* a place to collect waste paper, a storage depot for non-job sundries, or a flat surface on which to stack items you want to remember. One time-management consultant kept a close time log on an executive with a stacked desk and found that he spent over two hours daily looking for information on the top of his desk.

It is said there is no such thing as time management, as time cannot be managed, but there is self-management. Time does not waste itself, it needs help. Most of us work hard to in order to reap the benefits life has to offer. Consider how you can get the greatest return on your investment of time and energy. Strive to work less and accomplish more, but do not demand perfection from yourself. There will never be enough time for everything. But you can do a little less a little better.

KEY POINTS

➤ Keep tidy.
➤ Get organised.
➤ Plan your day.
➤ Clarify objectives.
➤ Group tasks.
➤ Do not procrastinate.
➤ Break up tasks.
➤ Always have something to read with you.
➤ Do difficult tasks when you are fresh; routine tasks when less so.
➤ Avoid perfectionism.
➤ Reduce interruptions.
➤ Learn to say 'no'.
➤ Reward yourself.
➤ Discard anything that you cannot influence or which does not affect your working life.

FURTHER READING

Adair J. *Effective Time Management: how to save time and spend it wisely*. Revised ed. Pan; 2009.

Alindina S. *Mindfulness for Dummies*. John Wiley & Sons; 2010.

Allen D. *Getting Things Done: how to achieve stress-free productivity* [paperback]. Piatkus; 2002.

De Mare G. *101 Ways to Protect Your Job: a handbook on how to handle your most valuable single asset – your job: advice from experts*. McGraw-Hill; 1984.

Kabat-Zinn J. *Full Catastrophe Living: how to cope with stress, pain and illness using Mindfulness meditation*. Piatkus; 2001.

Leboeuf M. *Working Smart: how to accomplish more in half the time*. Warner Books; 1998.

Turla PA, Hawkins KL. Time stretch. *Company Magazine*. 1983; **11**: 64–5.

Willson R, Branch R. *Cognitive Behaviour Therapy for Dummies*. John Wiley & Sons; 2006.

CHAPTER 15

Goal setting and change management

In this final chapter, we look at how to use your advanced communication and assertiveness skills to develop your leadership skills in planning, setting goals and managing change.

Anyone working in the health sector has had to learn to adapt, and learn fast. Careers are reshaped; additional responsibilities are accepted; the work changes in both style and content. Good management is proactive rather than reactive, so it is anticipated that those who will succeed will be those who have actively prepared for change – change is unsuccessful when it has been improvised and forced rather than planned. There is no magic formula for change management, but there are some clear themes, which include having a clear sense of direction, strong lines of communication, clear feedback from service users and robust performance management systems.

One of the early lessons of the 'best value' regime in local government, and more recent imposed changes, has been that many public sectors lack even the most basic data necessary to inform change management, and, as recent attempts to develop economic procurement for NHS supplies show, poor strategic sense.

To develop, people and organisations need to be experimental, creative, flexible and prepared to take risks. They need to keep informed of and measure and monitor trends and developments within their profession, and be in a position to assess changes and developments in attitudes and behaviour of competitors and society.

MANAGING CHANGE

Change is an inescapable part of our working lives, and yet most people resist change. We need to think broadly about change, and consider the following.

➤ What is change?
➤ Why do we need to change?
➤ How can we overcome resistance to change?
➤ How can we manage change and set goals?

Change is a constant in the workplace and world: to survive – and grow – we must adjust to change. Change is also messy, and risky. Just when you think you have arrived, you find you have hardly begun. Change is the key to progress, but we resist it because people react differently to change and change can be unsettling. It pays to be proactive, since if we assume no change, or try to escape it, our choices will be harsher. We need to adapt to a turbulent world. We need to be less passive and embrace change, and take part in setting the goals, as then we are empowered to alter our own futures. We have already seen changes operating in our careers, our pay, our pensions. There is a movement from hierarchical relationships towards procedures which encourage staff to work in flexible groups of equals. Work is no longer permanent and long term, and reward is more closely allied to achievement.

Change has to be managed and, as with any management process, it needs to be understood before it can be managed. We need to understand:

➤ how to plan for change
➤ how to implement change
➤ how to evaluate change.

Within this, we need to identify both the future that we desire and some of the forces driving change, plus our own reactions to change and the size and shape of the work to be done.

Step 1: Understanding the need for change

Everyone in healthcare should prepare themselves personally and professionally for change, as it is both fundamental to progress and necessary for survival. The NHS is not alone in facing big challenges. With yet another reorganisation we are looking at enormous changes in our working styles and job brief. GP practices are currently participating in major organisational change as they prepare to become small businesses operating within a consortium instead of in isolation. Hospitals are becoming stand-alone businesses; community trusts are breaking up into commissioning bodies or provider units; staff are having to skill up on their understanding of marketing and selling/trading services. In management, change is traditionally seen as common, rapid and huge in its effects. The public sector is no longer exempt.

It is not only management and the perceptions of their role that needs to change. Good communication within the workplace and organisation will be increasingly important. People will need to be kept informed and abreast of changes in policy and workload. New ideas must be regularly discussed and information shared, and new techniques must be tried out where appropriate. Everyone should be encouraged to raise issues affecting their work, and must indicate as soon as possible if accepted practice is inappropriate. Innovation and adaptability are becoming part of everyday life. It goes without saying that at this stage you need to keep abreast of, and not, all the positive reasons for the change, to counter the resistance you will face on your journey.

Step 2: Understanding resistance

Workplace change is always problematic and challenging to staff and management. It presents dilemmas and conflict:

➤ the need to experiment versus the need to be right
➤ the need to manage the present versus manage the change
➤ managing uncertainty versus certainty
➤ the balance between necessary bureaucracy versus innovation
➤ finally, what to focus on – external changes or internal changes.

There are no simple answers. Balances need to be struck, without compromising principles. We need to understand that resistance to change is often the expression of insecurity and fear: it exposes people to uncertainty and may alter work patterns for the worse. It is therefore more acceptable when the objectives and application are understood and do not offer a threat to security.

Such primitive anxieties sometimes lead organisations to construct particular routines and procedures that ultimately sabotage the very tasks they are required to carry out. Group practices, and individual burn out, lead people to become increasingly reluctant to care for patients. The study we looked at in Chapter 13,[1] which found that nurses experienced enormous emotional difficulties in working with dying patients, identified a number of uncomfortable working practices such as strict routines and division of labour; the idealisation of the professional, 'detached' nurse untouched by the death of a patient; the identification of patients by number rather than by name; the reduction in responsibility via delegation to superiors; and the avoidance of change.

These practices, while serving to reduce anxiety at both an organisational and a personal level, paradoxically reduced the nurses' emotional investment and satisfaction in relationships with their patients. Inhibition of the nurses' capacities and creative energies led to high levels of doubt and job dissatisfaction, which in turn led to a rapid and destabilising staff turnover at the hospital. This then further undermined the development of close and effective working relationships, which could have gone some way to offset the level of anxiety within the institution.

It is difficult to instigate change in organisations that are in the grip of such primitive defence systems. These are the very organisations that are least

---

1 Menzies Lyth I. Social systems as a defence against anxiety. *Human Relations*. 1959; **13**: 95–121. In: Rizq R. IATP, anxiety and envy: a psychoanalytic view of primary care mental health services today. *British Journal of Psychotherapy*. 2011; **27**(1): 37–55.

willing to appreciate the magnitude of their institutional problems and are consequently least able to undertake meaningful social change. We need to take care that we do not become so focused on our own needs, and that of the organisation, that the reasons we entered medicine are lost. We need to find working practices that meet the patient's need in order to regain emotional satisfaction with the work itself.

What individual resistance to change do we know about?

Reasons not to change
- ➤ Habit   Inconvenience   Own (biased) view of situation
- ➤ Loss of individualisation   Cost of change   Threat to own power base   Financial implications   Fear of the unknown
- ➤ Security is bedded in the past

EXERCISE 1

What are your own reasons not to change?

'I don't have the time.'
'We tried it five years ago and it didn't work.'
'Everyone will blame me if it doesn't work.'
'It's not in the plan.'
'I'm scared.'

Medical representatives have a secret code that classifies doctors. As a manager or colleague, it is worth considering how you best communicate change to each personality 'type'; see where you think you fit.

EXERCISE 2

- ➤ **Hares:** progressive, adventurous, believe in professional development and best practice. In selling to the hare, emphasise medicine and the patient, and show best evidence.
- ➤ **Dinosaurs:** reactionary, dissatisfied, resistant to change, old-fashioned. To support through change: show deference and respect, give support and sympathy.
- ➤ **Sheep:** conservative, traditional, conscientious, caring, avoid risk. In supporting, show respect, emphasise that this behaviour is standard, normal practice.

➤ **Wolves:** entrepreneurs; active, energetic, ambitious. They delegate responsibility and love change. Wolves do not need support but encouragement: emphasise any dynamic aspects of change and the benefits to the practitioners and organisation.

How do you react to change? Do you feel confident and excited or uncertain and frightened? Good managers manage the change process by acknowledging the uncomfortable side of change, as well and putting in place systems to cope with the turbulence.

Step 3: Identify the need for change
➤ Stay alert to the need for change.
➤ Consider where you are now.
➤ Consider where you want to be.

Step 4: Plan for change
Effective change needs careful planning. Any change in the workplace will affect everyone, and they may feel threatened. At this stage you need to identify who will be opposed and therefore not assist, who will not oppose but still not assist, and, to gain support, find out who will want it to happen, and make it happen. Recognise where there is agreement and conflict, and examine your own and staff training needs.

EXERCISE 3
Chart who you need to involve, highlighting those who will support and challenge the change, by placing stakeholders on a mind map, or as spokes around the hub of a wheel.[2]

---

2 Turrill T. *Change and Innovation in the NHS Management Series 10*. Institute of Health Service Management; 1986.

Moving premises

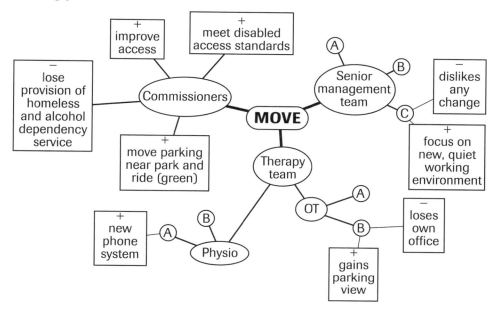

Step 5: Make the change, and make it successful

Experiment. Be dynamic. Change is successful when it has been preceded by other successful changes, and you have a clear set of cultural/organisational beliefs. You need to take charge, and to demonstrate that you have the energy, confidence and commitment to carry it through. Successful change is organic and dynamic, and involves innovation and ice-breaking. Leaders of change have passion, vision, a clear strategy, and are driven to manage the change.

Pointers to assist you in managing the change process:
➤ allow for a period of transition
➤ seek commitment and support
➤ seek out role models
➤ problem solve
➤ break things into steps: what needs to be done, when, by whom
➤ monitor your progress
➤ share your vision, your fundamental beliefs
➤ be honest with yourself
➤ listen to and understand the negatives
➤ acknowledge the history of organising things in a certain way, so any changes can be put on trial to see whether they work
➤ use your supporters' energy, enthusiasm and lead
➤ preserve as many of the existing benefits as possible

➤ make people aware of the inevitable losses as well as the gains
➤ involve staff in identifying the need for change, and planning the new
➤ provide facts to avoid rumour and uncertainty
➤ provide re-assurance
➤ communicate – keep an open door and an open mind.

Be aware of the effects of too much stress, and the effects of speedy change:

Shock ⟶ Defensive withdrawal ⟶ Acknowledgement ⟶ Adaptation

Allow for, and accommodate, these feelings, and respond to them by encouraging those affected to seek support if necessary.

Change can be both painful and unacceptable to those who are not 'change masters'. Some pertinent observations on how not to manage partnership change in the 1990s from the chief executive officer of a community health council involved in local consultations about local strategic issues[3] are shown below. The ideas are still relevant now.

How not to manage change
➤ Assume everyone will understand and accept the need for change straight away.
➤ Do not explain immediately, openly and clearly what you want to do and why.
➤ Allow time for rumours to circulate in order to increase anxiety and instability among the workforce and service users, and let these rumours reach the press before releasing your definitive plan.
➤ Be surprised and hurt when other groups attack or question your intentions: regard all resistance as an unfortunate obstacle to be overcome.
➤ If people express concerns which conflict with your own, console yourself with the thought that:
  – they are troublemakers and not representative
  – they cannot understand that what you want to do is the best thing
  – there are Luddites in every age who are always going to dislike change however necessary or desirable it is.
➤ Do not base your plans on accurate information and predictions.
➤ Always let your timescale slip for release of plans and their implementation – this ensures lack of impetus.
➤ Do not allow time for effective consultation: ask people their opinions and then take no notice of them.
➤ Never answer letters of query from outside interested parties. This makes people feel powerless and unheard.

---

3   Pattison S. Masters of change. *Health Service Journal.* 1991 Oct 31. p. 23.

➤ If you have to respond in some way, do so late so that they can make no use of any information you may provide.

➤ If you have to deal directly with angry interested parties, appear to take their concerns seriously, then get on with the real business of managing change. Do not allow their concerns to influence you – this could cloud your vision and might give them delusions of power.

➤ Reserve all initiatives for yourself – this also increases your power while enhancing the powerless of others – keep them guessing!

➤ Be economical with the truth about the reasons for change. Do not, for example, tell people that you are effectively making cuts because you do not have enough money. Tell them instead that what you are doing is best for them.

➤ Leave the future of the workforce vague. This destabilises people at a personal level and hopefully quite a lot of them will seek employment elsewhere, leaving more space and less opposition for the change you desire.

Clearly, if these attitudes and practice are applied, service users and workers will be effectively alienated and resistance to change will increase.

Step 6: Monitor and evaluate

Check that you have accomplished what you set out to do. Should the change be abandoned or adjusted? Talk to your team and find out. During the period of change, keep routine work under control so there is time to innovate and implement the new ways of working. It has been said that managers must view change and innovation as opportunities to seize rather than as threats to fear. We will only learn to master change when we encourage, welcome and incorporate it into our personal and professional lifestyle. Those who do not fear change grow, learn and continue to develop.

GOAL SETTING AND ORGANISATIONAL CHANGE

Goals can be personal ('Will I have my house in the country in 10 years time?', 'Will I get S into the school I want?') and professional ('Where will I be sitting in this organisation within five years?', 'How can I best lead the team through this change?', 'How can I manage my time better so I fit in my 20 contacts a week?'). We all need goals as they provide a basis for objectives, planning and control. They also help to develop individual commitment, reduce uncertainty in decision making and focus our direction.[4] As we know, we need the goals to tell us where to go, and the objectives to tell us how to get there.

---

4   Kast F, Rosenzweig J. *Organisation and Management: a systems and contingency approach.* 4th revised ed. McGraw-Hill; 1985.

What stops us from achieving goals? Achieving can only happen with good organisation and planning ahead. There are problems with setting NHS targets because of the sheer size of the organisation, and the fact that most problems in our resources and services are highly complex, with interrelated problems and opportunities, a fast-moving and unpredictable environment, and multiple interest groups. Many people have an interest in the target solution, and all will have different opinions, biases and interests. Different parts of the system have different problems, as each organisation is stand-alone and is structured and works very differently. Consider the aims, objectives, goals and service delivery of acute units, community and mental health trusts, with their limited year budgets and constant change imposed, compared with NHS management bodies such as strategic health authorities or commissioning groups. Here, change traditionally has been slower, more ponderous, but easier to plan and manage over time. Or primary care, where the ambulance service and A&E, for example, work reactively, so the ethos and culture is to manage reactively. Hence, change may be harder to plan for, implement and manage.

Managing the change and preventing failure

1 Plan the change

Chaos and disruption are common features when change is unplanned, and this creates additional stress, individually and throughout the team. In order to minimise and manage the risk of failure, even small teams can learn to address the major strategic issues and not simply concentrate on the operational management issues. Managers need to:
➤ map their environment
➤ understand the core purpose of their business
➤ paint a vision of their future.

Not all visions will be compatible. Whoever takes on the management role needs to assist the process of agreement within the senior management team/ partnership to define mutually acceptable aims. If personal and organisational goals are met and integrated, a stronger sense of identity will be developed and people will feel valued.

2 Team work

Failure occurs when goals have not been set and agreed/'owned' by the entire team. Ideas must be discussed and agreed before implementation. Change is difficult to manage at the best of times, but unless everyone is part of this type of discussion, sabotage is common.
➤ Find out the level of commitment, and allocate the responsibilities fairly.
➤ Talk through your ideas with interested stakeholders first.
➤ Check the viability of the plan first with your sponsors.

3   Manage conflict

We now know that conflict is a normal, and inevitable, reality of management and organisational behaviour. Remember that everyone has different needs, expectations, differences and attributes, then discuss where the conflict lies. Make the process mutual and participative, and try not to judge.

4   Manage the change through goal setting

You will never regret any positive move you make, however small. What you certainly will regret is not trying. People who never make mistakes, never make anything. Here we review some of the guidelines set out in Chapter 4 of my sister book, *Developing Assertiveness Skills for Health and Social Care Professionals*, where we used the principles of motivational interviewing to set goals and manage the change process for patients and clients. Personal, professional and management goals should be SMART.

➤ Specific, precise.
➤ Measurable (cost, quality, quantity, timeliness).
➤ Achievable within the timescale.
➤ Realistic (provide a challenge, stretch the employee).
➤ Timely (set a timeline that will guide your progress).
➤ Jointly established, not imposed.
➤ Broken down into objectives.
➤ Planned: indicate priorities (must do, could do), subject to a deadline.
➤ Continually updated.
➤ Checked for success.

If a particular task or goal is important enough, it is usually achieved, irrespective of all the obstacles and difficulties. The art of good management is identifying which goals are important, and achieving them using the minimum possible resources and without unnecessary stress. Develop positive and proactive thinking. Here are some tried and tested methods used by counsellors, trainers and coaches which may support you in achieving your aim. They can be used for both personal change/goal setting and managing professional changes. If you find it hard to set goals, be creative – use these ideas to assist you. Copy each exercise and complete one for any professional issues, one for personal development and one for your work-related issues.

5   Audit your success

EXERCISE 4

Get organised. If you find personal organisation difficult, complete the chart in Appendix A.

Then seek out the possible causes for poor organisation, and solve the problem.

?

➤ Lack of goals – write them down.

➤ Confusion in priorities – put first things first.

➤ Unrealistic time estimates – allow more time; allow for interruptions.

➤ Impatience with detail – take time to get it right.

➤ Manage by crisis – distinguish between urgent/important.

➤ Over commitment – delegate more.

➤ Knowledge explosion – read selectively.

➤ Over surveillance of subordinates – look to results, not detail.

➤ Refusal to delegate – accept that delegation is vital.

➤ Enjoyment of socialising – do it elsewhere; hold stand-up conferences.

➤ Indecision – make decisions with incomplete facts.

➤ Lack of confidence in the fact – improve your fact-finding procedures.

➤ Fear of the consequences of a mistake – use mistakes as your learning process.

➤ Fear of subordinates' inadequacy – train, allow mistakes; replace if necessary.

Another way of working on goals is to identify your current position.

Write the numbers 1 to 10 across the page: 1 is very negative, 10 is very positive. Circle the number that describes how you currently feel about your situation. This gives a statement of where you are to start working.

EXERCISE 5

If your goal is a more personal one, and you wish to, for example, become more assertive in managing your team, try the following.

Goals	Personal Strengths	Challenges	Development skills	Achievements

Complete this using the following guidelines.

Goals

Goals are the foundation stones. Make these positive: something you want to gain, not something you want to get rid of. Describe a goal, not a problem.

Personal strengths

Concentrate on your strengths, not your weaknesses. Do not downgrade your strengths. Believe you are worthy of what you want to achieve. Listing your strengths is a good way to focus on what you have to offer.

Immediate challenges/blocks/problems

Focus on problems that directly affect you – do not list problems that blame or involve other people. You cannot think or make goals for other people, only for yourself, so do not write: 'To get X to work harder.' Although your goal may well involve your X, you cannot think or make goals for them, only for yourself. Consider the problem from another angle: is there a way you can accommodate this worker? What are his or her strengths? How can this deficit challenge you less? This gives you command over the situation, and you have more control over solving it.

Development skills

This is an area you can develop and improve. Listing these is a great way to focus on the ways you can move forward. You are recognising that it takes two to communicate, and that you will take responsibility for the part you play. You might write 'Learn to listen more', or 'Improve how I give feedback'.

Achievements

List achievements you are proud of, positively: instead of 'I always fail at any new training I try to do', try 'At least I completed that training'. Other positive statements: 'I found the strength to leave a bad job and look for a good one', 'I am always willing to tackle problems and take risks'. Your achievements list is a great prompt to move you forward, because it makes you ask yourself the right questions, and to keep you positive and solution-oriented.

➤ What have I learnt from this?
➤ How have I progressed?
➤ What have I gained?
➤ How would I do things differently next time?

Finding the solution

The solution is always there, within you, although it may be hidden at the moment. Tease it out. Keep the focus on your own place in the problem. Ask yourself positive, self-focused and solution-focused questions: 'How can I ask questions in a way that X doesn't find threatening?' Keep asking yourself the right questions: 'How can I make this work for me?', 'How can I turn this situation around?'

Try these exercises, with a workplace flavour.

EXERCISE 6

Thought shower. Storm some solutions to long standing problems.

Then write down any that, in retrospect, you feel would work.

Write down those that you would not consider.

Are there any left over that you are not sure about? Do not dismiss them. Make a note of them here and come back to them at a later date.

> **Write or draw the consequences** of both problem and some of the solutions you are considering. If drawing, use symbols such as animals or a situation – a ski run, a boat race – to place yourself and others at the heart of the solution.

EXERCISE 7

If you feel at variance with your workplace culture, take time to list your personal core values. Living in conflict with our own inner values can lead to unhappiness, frustration and blocks. Becoming aware of your values and prioritising them helps you to reassess your goals.

1   Start by making a list of 10 values that you feel are important to you. Some common examples include: love, security, respect, money, achievement, health, success, ambition, freedom, integrity, compassion, independence, family, children, travel, trust.

2   Next, try to put your own values in order, from 1 to 10. This can be difficult, and you may need to rework your list a few times before you feel it really reflects how you think and feel. Once you have done that, look at what the list is telling you. For example, if security, commitment and loyalty are high on your list, and you are working on short-term contracts, you are behaving

in opposition to your values, and it will never make you happy. If freedom, independence and achievement are high on your list, you will need to be in a job that can give these qualities.

3   Compare this list with your life now, or how you are planning your life. Are you living your life as you should? Are you working in the right organisation? Do your values clash?

EXERCISE 8

Think of a solution to a problem. The items can be as large or small as you wish – use them to form a checklist of things done/to do.

EXERCISE 9

Goal analysis enables you to break down such instructions or goals into specific actions. These can then be used to measure how well the requirements are met, to audit qualitative criteria.

1   First, clarify your goal. The question 'How do people respond when they are made to feel welcome?' might produce a list such as:

happy
comfortable
satisfied
approving
appreciated
amiable.

2   Check each item for relevance and importance. For example, you might discard 'amiable' as being unimportant, and 'happy' as being irrelevant as unhappy people can still be made to feel welcome.

3   Having established how you would like people to feel in order for this goal to be met, next write down any action which would contribute to this, then identify the behaviour.

4   Having identified the behaviour that produces the required results, you may wish to set a specific target for that behaviour to be repeated, for example: 'Receptionists to alert patients of the appointment delay time every hour.' Aim to measure quality as well as quantity.

At times you may find that your attempts to analyse a certain goal get bogged down. You may end up chasing a different goal or even giving up the analysis. This does not necessarily mean that you are doing anything wrong. You will find out which goals are unnecessary, inappropriate or elusive. This method of goal analysis enables you to measure, to a greater or lesser degree, your achievements in meeting goals which are difficult to quantify. Those that can be checked against a graph or spreadsheet are simpler but no less important; it is essential for regular reviews to be conducted to monitor the state and progress of all the goals.

SETTING OBJECTIVES AND TARGETS

Objectives, like goals, should be:

➤ measurable
➤ realistic and achievable
➤ time bound.

Note also any critical success factors, and build in a system for monitoring whether you have achieved your objectives. Use the following table as a template.

Objective/ target	How will you measure success?	Who responsible?	Date for action	Cost	Achieved by

Here is a selection of the aims one manager set for herself.

➤ Improve communication with staff.
➤ Select different chair for meetings.
➤ Need to learn more about working strategically not operationally.
➤ Delegate more.
➤ Need to improve financial management skills and develop appropriate management systems.

How does this fit into a plan? Once you have identified your priorities, and have costed them, stage them, marking each target with an aim (what the plan is) and an objective (how to map the outcome).

➤ Detail your targets for the year to come.
➤ Note how success will be measured once the object has been achieved,
➤ Note who is responsible for achieving it by when, using basic *Who *Why *What *Where *When headings. Note the cost, if any, of your plan, and when you hope to achieve it by.
➤ Be specific and clear about your objectives.

Then consider how these aims should be prioritised, how success will be measured once the object has been achieved, and who is responsible for achieving it, by when. With the date, cost and achieved date noted, you have a complete record of the process. See Appendix B if you tend to procrastinate.

PLANNING

What are you currently doing towards meeting your present goal?
What do you plan to do next year?

Good planning is essential to a smooth-running, communicating organisation. The *process* of planning enables you to:
➤ see clearly where you are at present
➤ clarify some of the wider issues facing you or your organisation
➤ firm up any new proposals
➤ evaluate yourself and the organisation
➤ provide a statement of intent for interested stakeholders
➤ formulate goals
➤ identify the action needed to achieve these goals
➤ identify resources required in terms of skills, activity and finance
➤ anticipate ahead
➤ ensure the negotiation of the best possible funding.

How do we plan?
➤ Identify the problem.
➤ Collect the data to quantify the problem.
➤ Analyse the problem.
➤ Organise and co-ordinate a plan of action.
➤ Implement.
➤ Review.
➤ Monitor.

Good planning involves strong leadership skills: delegation, objectivity, realism, flexibility and logical thinking. Plans need to be widely communicated: they need everyone's involvement and team work. Plans need time to think out and implement. Prior planning is a management skill that helps to prevent poor performance. What follows are some tried and tested planning supports.

Use a chart to plan

If you are changing your computer system moving premises, for example, try planning the stages using a chart, with the goals on the vertical axis, and the timescale on the horizontal:

	By	1 Aug	7 Aug	14 Aug	21 Aug
Contact solicitors					
Alert and publicise to stakeholders					
Change publicity					
Plan removal					
Sell unwanted equipment					
Confirm change to computer company					
Confirm removal date					
Contact utilities					

Projects

When writing a project brief, take the reader step by step through the process:
➤ a proposal
➤ detail of the project
➤ ways of evaluating the performance.

It is important to ensure consistency and focus through the project's life cycle. One way of doing this is to prioritise goals and objectives with specific indicators: must do, could do. You must do something if the risk to the practice or project is high, but not if the impact is low. This example looks at the risk of not managing the risk of a burglary within a practice.

Risk	Probability	Impact
Of burglary if practice unsecured	High	High: insurance/disruption costs
PCT will not reimburse	Medium	Low: practice will pay
Threat to staff- duplication	High	High
No real financial gain	High	High

Audit your success

Having defined your goals and planned their implementation, the next step is to audit your success in meeting them.

SUMMARY

Having completed this chapter, and worked through the exercises in the book, you should now have a sense of improved self-awareness and self-knowledge. The book aimed to develop your individual strengths and talents and help you identify and improve your potential and personal autonomy. Assertiveness helps us fulfil aspirations. Personal development is also about establishing identity; developing competence, purpose and integrity and mature interpersonal relationships; managing emotions; and achieving interdependence.

You will now, I hope, understand what assertiveness is and the skills needed to become assertive. You will have explored some of the personal and professional challenges, broadening your understanding of other people and how they operate. You will have learned how to manage conflict and aggression, and how to manage difficult colleagues with understanding, expertise and compassion. We addressed the foundations of good communication and the need to understand what your organisation and team really looks like. We have developed an understanding of ourselves: our need to be assertive, our motivations, personality, how we work within a team. We have explored how to use assertion skills to develop professionally and personally: in planning and managing life to help make it stress free through goal setting, time and change management.

You will have learnt how you can apply assertiveness skills to develop yourself, and your relationships with your colleagues at work. You will have learnt how to manage yourself more effectively, and, hopefully, how to be a more informed and effective worker within the ever-changing care sector.

If you know yourself and understand others better, you are more likely to be able to take control of your life, and to live it actively rather than passively. As you take on more responsibility, a different kind of respect is demanded, which has intellectual, spiritual, personal, psychological and emotional implications. You will be ready to move on and up.

List all the things you aim to achieve over your lifetime.
List those you could reasonably achieve within 10 years.
List those you will achieve this year.

KEY POINTS

➤ Good management is proactive rather than reactive; so it is anticipated that those who succeed will be those who have actively prepared for change.

➤ 'Good' change occurs when there is a clear sense of strategy and direction, strong lines of communication, clear feedback from service users and robust performance management systems.

➤ To develop, people and organisations need to be experimental, creative, flexible and prepared to take risks. They need to keep informed of, measure and monitor trends and developments within their profession, and be in a position to assess changes and developments in attitudes and behaviour of competitors, patients and society.

➤ Change is a constant in the workplace and world: to survive – and grow – we must adjust to change. We need to understand that resistance to change is often the expression of insecurity and fear as security is bedded in the past, so communication is vital. Allow for, and accommodate, these feelings, and respond to them by encouraging those affected to seek support.

➤ Change has to be managed and, as with any management process, it needs to be understood before it can be managed. We need to understand how to plan for, implement and evaluate it. We need to understand the forces driving change and our own reactions to it, and measure the size and shape of the work to be done.

➤ Change is always problematic because it presents dilemmas and conflict, so balances need to be struck, without compromising principles.

➤ Successful change is organic and dynamic, and involves innovation and ice-breaking. Leaders of change have passion, vision, a clear strategy, and are driven to manage the change.

➤ We all need goals as they provide a basis for objectives, planning and control. They also help to develop individual commitment, reduce uncertainty in decision making and focus our direction.

➤ There are problems with change within the NHS and social care because of the organisational size and complexity. Both are fast-moving and unpredictable environments, and contain multiple interest groups.

➤ Chaos and disruption are common features when change is unplanned, so managers need to map their environment, understand the core purpose of their business and paint a vision of their future. Goals have to be identified, analysed, and agreed by all stakeholders. Any conflict needs sensitive and active managing.

➤ Goal analysis means unpicking strengths, identifying immediate challenges/blocks/problems and development skills and achievements.

➤ Becoming aware of your core values and prioritising them helps you to assess your goals.

➤ List all the things you would like to achieve over your lifetime.
➤ List those you could reasonably achieve within 10 years.
➤ List those you will achieve this year.
➤ Audit your success.
➤ What are you currently doing towards meeting your present goal? What do you plan to do next year?

FURTHER READING

Audit Commission. *Change Here! Managing change to improve local services.* Audit Commission; 2001. Available at: http://archive.audit-commission.gov.uk/audit-commission/nationalstudies/localgov/Pages/changehere.aspx.html (accessed April 2013).

Belasen A. *Leading the Learning Organisation: communication and competencies for managing change.* SUNY Series in Human Communication Processes. State University of New York Press; 1999.

Cameron E, Green M. *Making Sense of Change Management: a complete guide to the models tools and techniques of organizational change.* Kogan Press; 2009.

Carter R, Martin JNT, Mayblin B, *et al. Systems, Management and Change: a graphic guide.* Paul Chapman Publishing Ltd/Open University; 1984.

Hayes J. *The Theory and Practice of Change Management.* 3rd ed. Palgrave Macmillan; 2010.

Herzberg F. *Motivation to Work.* Transaction Publishers; 1993.

Locke A, Latham G. *A Theory of Goal Setting and Task Performance.* Prentice-Hall; 1989.

Locke A, Latham G. *Goal Setting: a motivational technique that works.* Prentice Hall; 1984.

Newton R. *Managing Change Step by Step: all you need to build a plan and make it happen.* Pearson Business; 2007.

Harvard Business School Press. *Managing Change and Transition.* Harvard Business Essential. Harvard Business School Press; 2003.

APPENDIX A: PERSONAL ORGANISATION

For the factors below, circle the number that most represents your view of your organisation skills.

1	I am ruthless with paperwork. I only keep top priority paperwork for the time it is needed.	1	2	3	4	5	I have never thought about paperwork. I tend to keep all of it for too long.
2	I have now developed a desk organisation system based upon my top priority work.	1	2	3	4	5	My desk organisation system is haphazard; often it is non-existent.
3	Normally I can retrieve information quickly from my system.	1	2	3	4	5	I normally have to search a great deal for my information. Sometimes I lose essential pieces of information.
4	I use my desk for *working* on and I operate a *clear desk* policy.	1	2	3	4	5	I use my desk to *store* work on. I don't operate a *clear desk* policy.

		1	2	3	4	5	
5	When I am working on top priority work, I make sure that I will not be interrupted unless it is a top priority interruption.	1	2	3	4	5	When I am working on top priority work, I am often interrupted. I have difficulty in dealing with these interruptions.
6	I very rarely give *prior right* to an interruption.	1	2	3	4	5	Normally interruptions do take *prior right* over the work I am doing at the time.
7	In my work team we have established a code of practice on interruptions.	1	2	3	4	5	We have no code of practice for interruptions in my work team.
8	I always batch my phone calls into top and low priority.	1	2	3	4	5	I have no priority system for phone calls and I make them at any time during the day.
9	For top priority work, I never rely on being rung back. I make appointments to ring back again until I have the information.	1	2	3	4	5	For top priority work, I always ask the manager to ring me back if not available or if information is not available.
10	My opening line in a phone call is my name, purpose and action.	1	2	3	4	5	My opening line in a phone call is my name.
11	I often hold long phone conversations on top priority work in preference to a meeting.	1	2	3	4	5	I very rarely hold long phone conversations on top priority work. Meetings are preferable.
12	For much of my lower priority work, my secretary or subordinate will handle it directly.	1	2	3	4	5	I have not briefed my secretary or subordinates on handling lower priority work.

APPENDIX B: AVOIDING PROCRASTINATION

Successful approaches for difficult tasks

➤ Use the five-minute brainstorm: break the project down into smaller activities and write these down.
➤ Focus attention on the smaller, individual activities: Concentrate on the smaller, bit-sized pieces to avoid feeling overwhelmed.

➤ Block out an adequate length of time: do not start work just before lunch or meetings – it will only reinforce your negative feelings.

➤ Work when you are at your best: reserve quality time for important jobs and do the low payoff tasks after lunch and at other low times.

➤ Start each session with something easy: do anything to get going rather than nothing at all.

➤ Redefine the project: others may have ideas to simplify it. Remember: better to deliver a simple one on time than not deliver a complex one.

Successful approaches for long-term tasks

➤ Determine a realistic time commitment per week: better to set and stick to an hour a week than to set 10 hours and do nothing. Even the largest project will respond to steady progress.

➤ Specify tasks in advance: end each session by specifying the next session's work. This enables your subconscious to work on it and also makes it easier to get started next time.

➤ Establish a regular time for working on long-term projects: it will help to make it become a habit.

➤ Establish deadlines for intermediate progress points: set self-imposed deadlines for short-term activities which can be completed in a week or less.

➤ Switch to other aspects of the overall task: prevent boredom or frustration by working on different areas of the project.

➤ Avoid the activity trap: do not lose sight of the long-term goal.

➤ Limit the number of major projects: remember that routine activities will take up a large proportion of your time.

➤ Record your ongoing progress each week: any form of diary, calendar or graph can be used to show that you are making progress.

➤ Improve efficiency by grouping similar tasks.

➤ Break up tasks into manageable chunks.

➤ Make time work for you: always have something to read or work on with you.

➤ Reduce interruptions and time leaks: set aside chunks of quality time and use them profitably.

➤ Avoid perfectionism: it costs too much.

Index

CPD with Radcliffe

You can now use a selection of our books to achieve CPD (Continuing Professional Development) points through directed reading.

We provide a free online form and downloadable certificate for your appraisal portfolio. Look for the CPD logo and register with us at: **www.radcliffehealth.com/cpd**

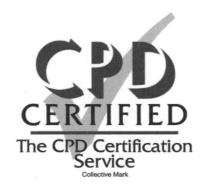